My Ultimate Keto Diet Cooking Guide

A Handful of New, Innovative and Delicious Keto Recipes for Women Over 50

Grace Studridge

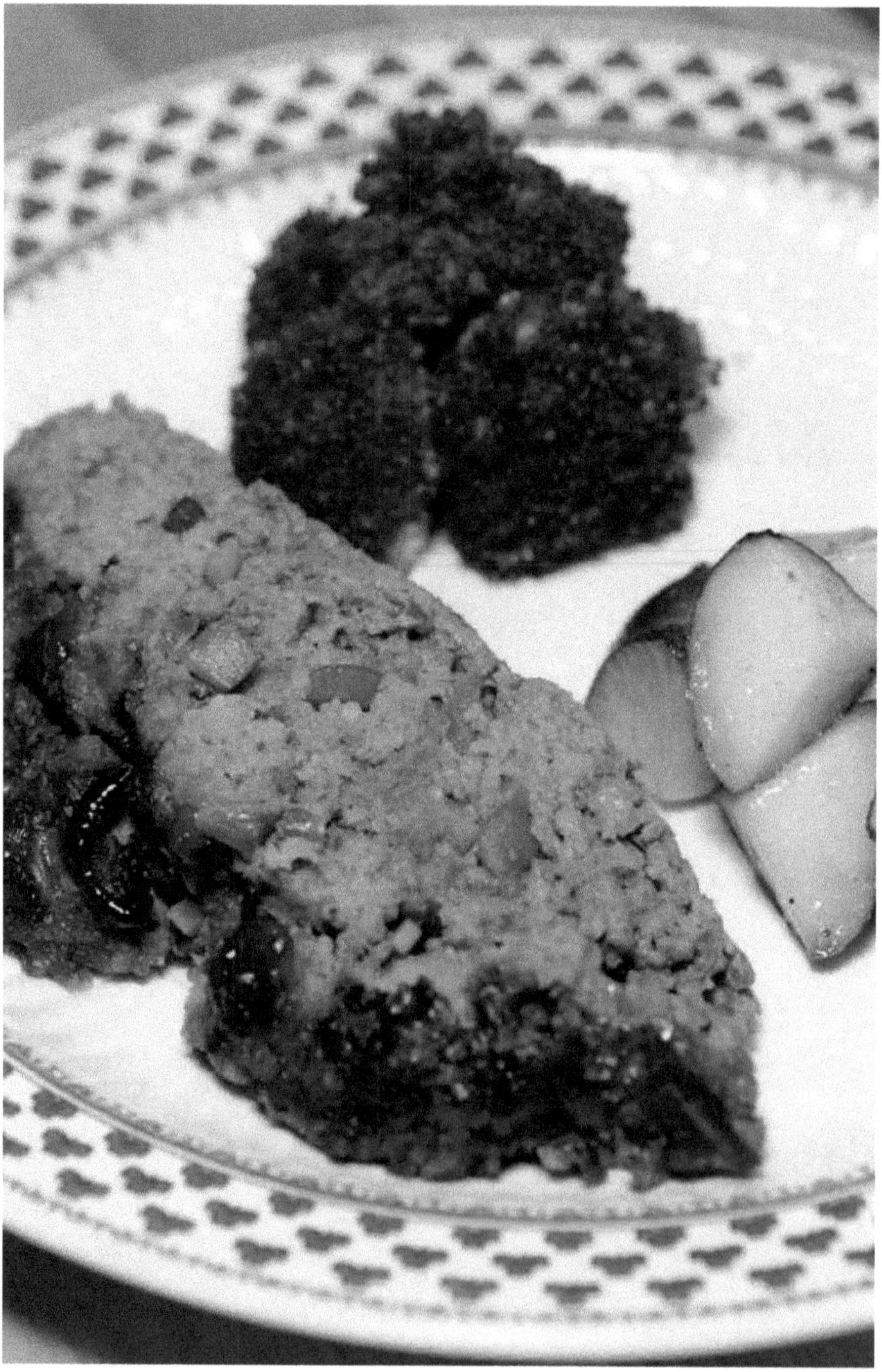

Readers acknowledge that the author is not engaging in the rendering of legal, financial, medical or professional advice. The content within this book has been derived from various sources. Please consult a licensed professional before attempting any techniques outlined in this book.

By reading this document, the reader agrees that under no circumstances is the author responsible for any losses, direct or indirect, which are incurred as a result of the use of information contained within this document, including, but not limited to, — errors, omissions, or inaccuracies.

TABLE OF CONTENTS

BEEF, PEPPER AND GREEN BEANS STIR-FRY 8

CHEESY MEATLOAF 10

ROAST BEEF AND VEGETABLE PLATE...............................12

STEAK AND CHEESE PLATE 14

GARLICKY STEAKS WITH ROSEMARY.................................16

FISH AND EGG PLATE 19

SESAME TUNA SALAD 21

KETO TUNA SANDWICH 22

TUNA MELT JALAPENO PEPPERS.......................................25

SMOKED SALMON FAT BOMBS...27

SALMON CUCUMBER ROLLS 29

BACON WRAPPED MAHI-MAHI..31

CHEESY GARLIC BREAD WITH SMOKED SALMON 33

SMOKED SALMON PASTA SALAD 35

TUNA SALAD PICKLE BOATS...37

SHRIMP DEVILED EGGS..39

HERB CRUSTED TILAPIA 40

TUNA STUFFED AVOCADO 42

GARLIC BUTTER SALMON...43

SALMON WITH GREEN BEANS..45

SALMON SHEET PAN..47

BACON WRAPPED SALMON..49

STIR-FRY TUNA WITH VEGETABLES................................51

CHILI-GLAZED SALMON 53

CARDAMOM SALMON...54

CREAMY TUNA, SPINACH, AND EGGS PLATES...............56

TUNA AND AVOCADO...57

BAKED FISH WITH FETA AND TOMATO.........................59

GARLIC OREGANO FISH 61

FISH AND SPINACH PLATE..62

FISH WITH KALE AND OLIVES.......................................64

MAHI-MAHI WITH CHILI LIME BUTTER 66

GINGER SESAME GLAZED SALMON...............................68

TUNA, DILL AND SPINACH CURRY BOWL 70

MUSHROOM WITH SALMON 71

TUNA SALAD CUCUMBER BOATS.................................73

SALMON WITH LIME BUTTER SAUCE 75

BLACKENED FISH WITH ZUCCHINI NOODLES................77

GARLIC PARMESAN MAHI-MAHI 79

SALMON WITH ROASTED VEGGIES 80

CHEESY BAKED MAHI-MAHI 82

ZUCCHINI NOODLES IN CREAMY SALMON SAUCE........84

WINTER COMFORT STEW 87

IDEAL COLD WEATHER STEW 89

WEEKEND DINNER STEW 91

MEXICAN PORK STEW..93

HUNGARIAN PORK STEW..96

YELLOW CHICKEN SOUP...98

CURRY SOUP..100

DELICIOUS TOMATO BASIL SOUP...103

30-DAY MEAL PLAN 105

Beef, Pepper and Green Beans Stir-fry

Preparation Time : 5 minutes;
Cooking Time : 18 minutes

 Servings : 2

Ingredients

- 6 oz ground beef
- 2 oz chopped green bell pepper
- 4 oz green beans
- 3 tbsp. grated cheddar cheese
- Seasoning:
- ½ tsp salt
- ¼ tsp ground black pepper
- ¼ tsp paprika

Directions:

1. Take a skillet pan, place it over medium heat, add ground beef and cook for 4 minutes until slightly browned.
2. Then add bell pepper and green beans, season with salt, paprika, and black pepper, stir well and continue cooking for 7 to 10 minutes until beef and vegetables have cooked through.
3. Sprinkle cheddar cheese on top, then transfer pan under the broiler and cook for 2 minutes until cheese has melted and the top is golden brown.

4. Serve.

Nutrition :
282.5 Calories; 17.6 g Fats; 26.1 g Protein; 2.9 g Net Carb; 2.1 g
Fiber;

Cheesy Meatloaf

Preparation Time : 5 minutes
Cooking Time : 4 minutes

Servings : 2

Ingredients

- 4 oz ground turkey
- 1 egg
- 1 tbsp. grated mozzarella cheese
- ¼ tsp Italian seasoning
- ½ tbsp. soy sauce
- Seasoning:
- ¼ tsp salt
- 1/8 tsp ground black pepper

Directions:

1. Take a bowl, place all the ingredients in it, and stir until mixed.
2. Take a heatproof mug, spoon in prepared mixture and microwave for 3 minutes at high heat setting until cooked.
3. When done, let meatloaf rest in the mug for 1 minute, then take it out, cut it into two slices and serve.

Nutrition :

196.5 Calories; 13.5 g Fats; 18.7 g Protein; 18.7 g Net Carb; 0 g Fiber;

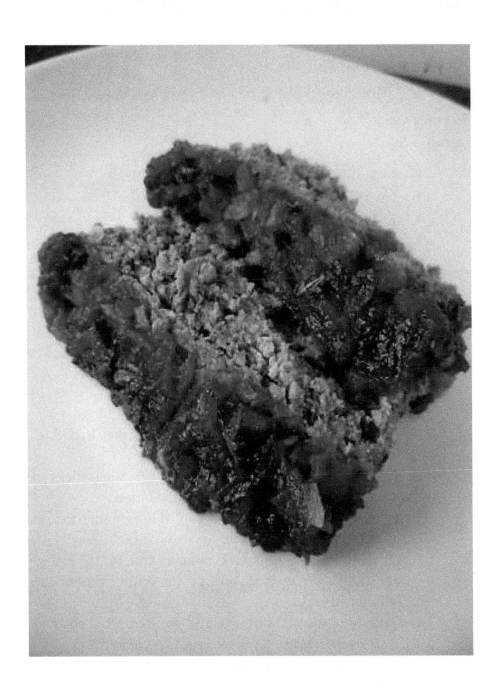

Roast Beef and Vegetable Plate

Preparation Time : 10 minutes
Cooking Time : 10 minutes;

Servings : 2

Ingredients

- 2 scallions, chopped in large pieces
- 1 ½ tbsp. coconut oil
- 4 thin slices of roast beef
- 4 oz cauliflower and broccoli mix
- 1 tbsp. butter, unsalted
- Seasoning:
- 1/2 tsp salt
- 1/3 tsp ground black pepper
- 1 tsp dried parsley

Directions:

1. Turn on the oven, then set it to 400 degrees F, and let it preheat.
2. Take a baking sheet, grease it with oil, place slices of roast beef on one side, and top with butter.
3. Take a separate bowl, add cauliflower and broccoli mix, add scallions, drizzle with oil, season with remaining salt and black pepper, toss until coated and then spread vegetables on the empty side of the baking sheet.
4. Bake for 5 to 7 minutes until beef is nicely browned and vegetables are tender-crisp, tossing halfway.
5. Distribute beef and vegetables between two plates and then serve.

Nutrition :

313 Calories; 26 g Fats; 15.6 g Protein; 2.8 g Net Carb; 1.9 g Fiber;

Steak and Cheese Plate

Preparation Time : 5 minutes;

Cooking Time : 10 minutes;

Servings : 2

Ingredients

- 1 green onion, chopped
- 2 oz chopped lettuce
- 2 beef steaks
- 2 oz of cheddar cheese, sliced
- ½ cup mayonnaise
- Seasoning:
- ¼ tsp salt
- 1/8 tsp ground black pepper
- 3 tbsp. avocado oil

Directions:

1. Prepare the steak, and for this, season it with salt and black pepper.
2. Take a medium skillet pan, place it over medium heat, add oil and when hot, add seasoned steaks, and cook for 7 to 10 minutes until cooked to the desired level.
3. When done, distribute steaks between two plates, add scallion, lettuce, and cheese slices.
4. Drizzle with remaining oil and then serve with mayonnaise.

Nutrition :

714 Calories; 65.3 g Fats; 25.3 g Protein; 4 g Net Carb; 5.3 g Fiber;

Garlicky Steaks with Rosemary

Preparation Time : 25 minutes
Cooking Time : 12 minutes;

Servings : 2

Ingredients

- 2 beef steaks
- 1/4 of a lime, juiced
- 1 ½ tsp garlic powder
- ¾ tsp dried rosemary
- 2 ½ tbsp. avocado oil
- Seasoning:
- ½ tsp salt
- ¼ tsp ground black pepper

Directions:

1. Prepare steaks, and for this, sprinkle garlic powder on all sides of steak.
2. Take a shallow dish, place 1 ½ tbsp. oil and lime juice in it, whisk until combined, add steaks, turn to coat and let it marinate for 20 minutes at room temperature.
3. Then take a griddle pan, place it over medium-high heat and grease it with remaining oil.
4. Season marinated steaks with salt and black pepper, add to the griddle pan and cook for 7 to 12 minutes until cooked to the desired level.
5. When done, wrap steaks in foil for 5 minutes, then cut into slices across the grain.

6. Sprinkle rosemary over steaks slices and then serve.

Nutrition :

213 Calories; 13 g Fats; 22 g Protein; 1 g Net Carb; 0 g Fiber;

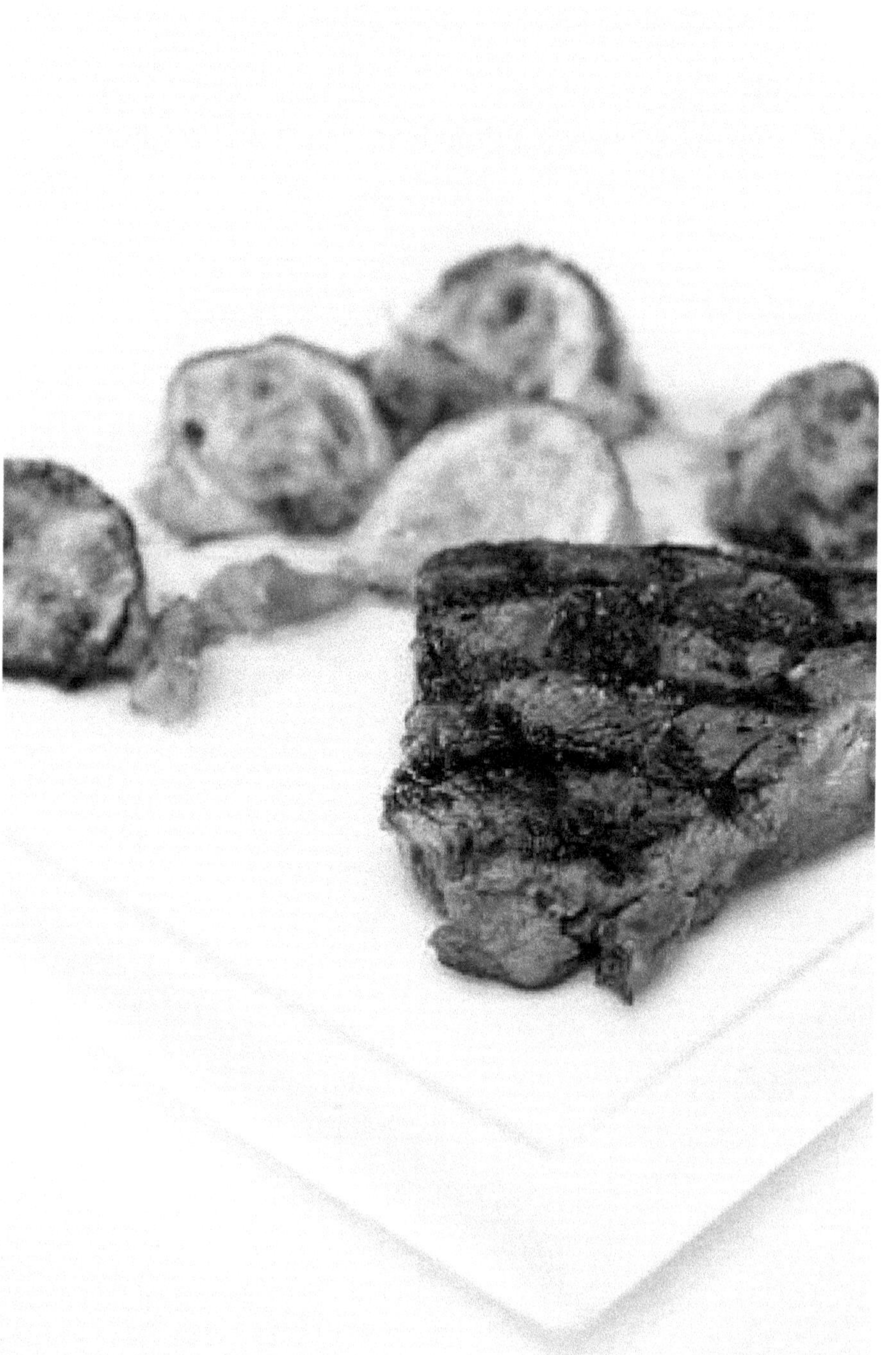

Fish and Egg Plate

Preparation Time : 5 minutes;

Cooking Time : 10 minutes;

Servings : 2

Ingredients

- 2 eggs
- 1 tbsp. butter, unsalted
- 2 pacific whitening fillets
- ½ oz chopped lettuce
- 1 scallion, chopped
- Seasoning:
- 3 tbsp. avocado oil
- 1/3 tsp salt
- 1/3 tsp ground black pepper

Directions:

1. Cook the eggs and for this, take a frying pan, place it over medium heat, add butter and when it melts, crack the egg in the pan and cook for 2 to 3 minutes until fried to desired liking.
2. Transfer fried egg to a plate and then cook the remaining egg in the same manner.
3. Meanwhile, season fish fillets with ¼ tsp each of salt and black pepper.
4. When eggs have fried, sprinkle salt and black pepper on them, then add 1 tbsp. oil into the frying pan, add fillets and cook for 4 minutes per side until thoroughly cooked.

5. When done, distribute fillets to the plate, add lettuce and scallion, drizzle with remaining oil, and then serve.

Sesame Tuna Salad

Preparation Time : 35 minutes

Cooking Time : 0 minutes;

Servings : 2

Ingredients

- 6 oz of tuna in water
- ½ tbsp. chili-garlic paste
- ½ tbsp. black sesame seeds, toasted
- 2 tbsp. mayonnaise
- 1 tbsp. sesame oil
- Seasoning:
- 1/8 tsp red pepper flakes

Directions:

1. Take a medium bowl, all the ingredients for the salad in it except for tuna, and then stir until well combined.
2. Fold in tuna until mixed and then refrigerator for 30 minutes.
3. Serve.

Nutrition:

322 Calories; 25.4 g Fats; 17.7 g Protein; 2.6 g Net Carb; 3 g Fiber;

Keto Tuna Sandwich

Preparation Time : 10 minutes
Cooking Time : 10 minutes;

Servings : 2

Ingredients

- 2 oz tuna, packed in water
- 2 2/3 tbsp. coconut flour
- 1 tsp baking powder
- 2 eggs
- 2 tbsp. mayonnaise
- Seasoning:
- 1/4 tsp salt
- 1/4 tsp ground black pepper

Directions:

1. Turn on the oven, then set it to 375 degrees F and let it preheat.
2. Meanwhile, prepare the batter for this, add all the ingredients in a bowl, reserving mayonnaise, 1 egg, and 1/8 tsp salt, and then whisk until well combined.
3. Take a 4 by 4 inches heatproof baking pan, grease it with oil, pour in the prepared batter and bake 10 minutes until bread is firm.
4. Meanwhile, prepare tuna and for this, place tuna in a medium bowl, add mayonnaise, season with remaining salt and black pepper, and then stir until combined.

5. When done, let the bread cool in the pan for 5 minutes, then transfer it to a wire rack and cool for 20 minutes.
6. Slice the bread, prepare sandwiches with prepared tuna mixture, and then serve.

Nutrition:
255 Calories; 17.8 g Fats; 16.3 g Protein; 3.7 g Net Carb; 3.3 g Fiber;

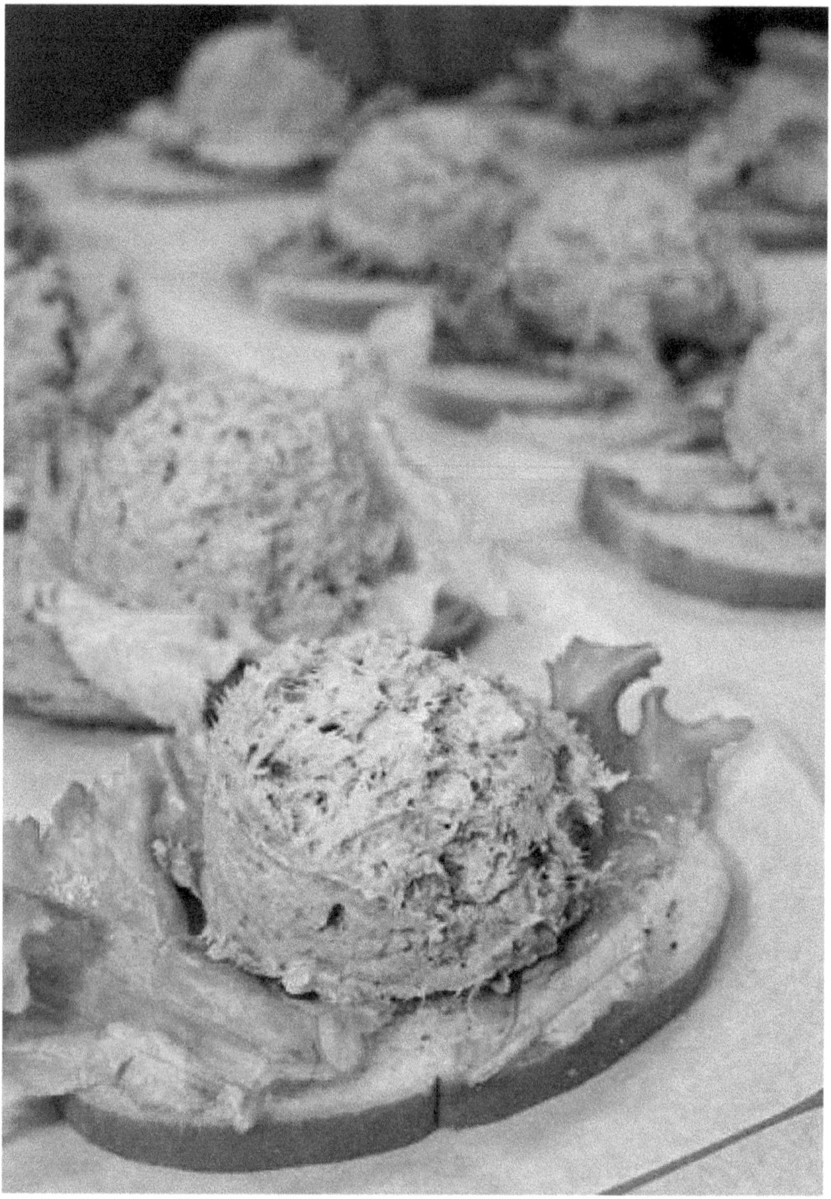

Tuna Melt Jalapeno Peppers

Preparation Time : 5 minutes

Cooking Time : 10 minutes;

Servings : 2

Ingredients

- 4 jalapeno peppers
- 1-ounce tuna, packed in water
- 1-ounce cream cheese softened
- 1 tbsp. grated parmesan cheese
- 1 tbsp. grated mozzarella cheese
- Seasoning:
- 1 tsp chopped dill pickles
- 1 green onion, green part sliced only

Directions:

1. Turn on the oven, then set it to 400 degrees F and let it preheat.
2. Prepare the peppers and for this, cut each pepper in half lengthwise and remove seeds and stem.
3. Take a small bowl, place tuna in it, add remaining ingredients except for cheeses, and then stir until combined.
4. Spoon tuna mixture into peppers, sprinkle cheeses on top, and then bake for 7 to 10 minutes until cheese has turned golden brown.
5. Serve.

Nutrition:

104 Calories; 6.2 g Fats; 7 g Protein; 2.1 g Net Carb; 1.1 g Fiber;

Smoked Salmon Fat Bombs

Preparation Time : 5 minutes

Cooking Time : 0 minutes;

Servings : 2

Ingredients

- 2 tbsp. cream cheese, softened
- 1 ounce smoked salmon
- 2 tsp bagel seasoning

Directions:

1. Take a medium bowl, place cream cheese and salmon in it, and stir until well combined.
2. Shape the mixture into bowls, roll them into bagel seasoning and then serve.

Nutrition :

65 Calories; 4.8 g Fats; 4 g Protein; 0.5 g Net Carb; 0 g Fiber;

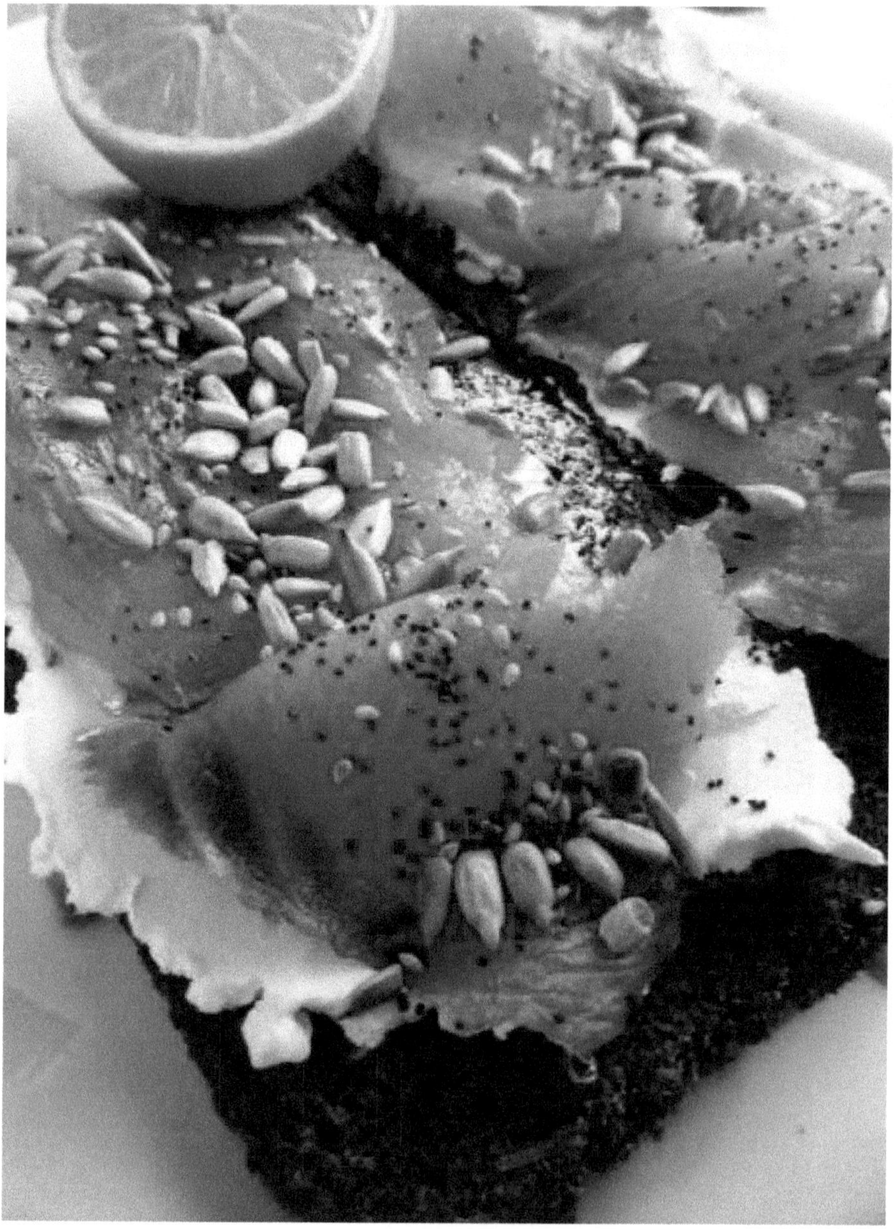

Salmon Cucumber Rolls

Preparation Time : 15 minutes;

Cooking Time : 0 minutes;

Servings : 2

Ingredients

- 1 large cucumber
- 2 oz smoked salmon
- 4 tbsp. mayonnaise
- 1 tsp sesame seeds
- Seasoning:
- ¼ tsp salt
- ¼ tsp ground black pepper

Directions:

1. Trim the ends of the cucumber, cut it into slices by using a vegetable peeler, and then place half of the cucumber slices in a dish.
2. Cover with paper towels, layer with remaining cucumber slices, top with paper towels, and let them refrigerate for 5 minutes.
3. Meanwhile, take a medium bowl, place salmon in it, add mayonnaise, season with salt and black pepper, and then stir until well combined.
4. Remove cucumber slices from the refrigerator, place salmon on one side of each cucumber slice, and then roll tightly.

5. Repeat with remaining cucumber, sprinkle with sesame seeds and then serve.

Nutrition:
269 Calories; 24 g Fats; 6.7 g Protein; 4 g Net Carb; 2 g Fiber;

Bacon Wrapped Mahi-Mahi

Preparation Time : 10 minutes

Cooking Time : 12 minutes;

Servings : 2

Ingredients

2 fillets of mahi-mahi

2 strips of bacon

½ of lime, zested

4 basil leaves

½ tsp salt

Seasoning:

½ tsp ground black pepper

1 tbsp. avocado oil

Directions:

1. Turn on the oven, then set it to 375 degrees F and let them preheat.
2. Meanwhile, season fillets with salt and black pepper, top each fillet with 2 basil leaves, sprinkle with lime zest, wrap with a bacon strip and secure with a toothpick if needed.
3. Take a medium skillet pan, place it over medium-high heat, add oil and when hot, place prepared fillets in it and cook for 2 minutes per side.
4. Transfer pan into the oven and bake the fish for 5 to 7 minutes until thoroughly cooked.

5. Serve.

Nutrition :

217 Calories; 11.3 g Fats; 27.1 g Protein; 1.2 g Net Carb; 0.5 g Fiber;

Cheesy Garlic Bread with Smoked Salmon

Preparation Time : 10 minutes
Cooking Time : 1 minute;

Servings : 2

Ingredients

- 4 tbsp. almond flour
- ½ tsp baking powder
- 2 tbsp. grated cheddar cheese
- 1 egg
- 2 oz salmon, cut into thin sliced
- Seasoning:
- 1 tbsp. butter, unsalted
- ¼ tsp garlic powder
- 1/8 tsp salt
- ¼ tsp Italian seasoning

Directions:

1. Take a heatproof bowl, place all the ingredients in it except for cheese and then stir by using a fork until well combined.
2. Fold in cheese until just mixed and then microwave for 1 minute at high heat setting until thoroughly cooked, else continue cooking for another 15 to 30 seconds.

3. When done, lift out the bread, cool it for 5 minutes and then cut it into slices.
4. Top each slice with salmon and then serve straight away

Nutrition :

233 Calories; 18 g Fats; 13.8 g Protein; 1.9 g Net Carb; 1.5 g Fiber;

Smoked Salmon Pasta Salad

Preparation Time : 10 minutes
Cooking Time : 0 minutes;

Servings : 2

Ingredients

- 1 zucchini, spiralized into noodles
- 4 oz smoked salmon, break into pieces
- 2 oz cream cheese
- 2 oz mayonnaise
- 2 oz sour cream
- Seasoning:
- 1/3 tsp salt
- ¼ tsp ground black pepper
- ¼ tsp hot sauce

Directions:

1. Take a medium bowl, place cream cheese in it, add mayonnaise, sour cream, salt, black pepper and hot sauce and stir until well combined.
2. Add zucchini noodles, toss until well coated and then fold in salmon until just mixed.
3. Serve.

Nutrition:

458 Calories; 38.7 g Fats; 15.4 g Protein; 6.1 g Net Carb; 1.7 g Fiber;

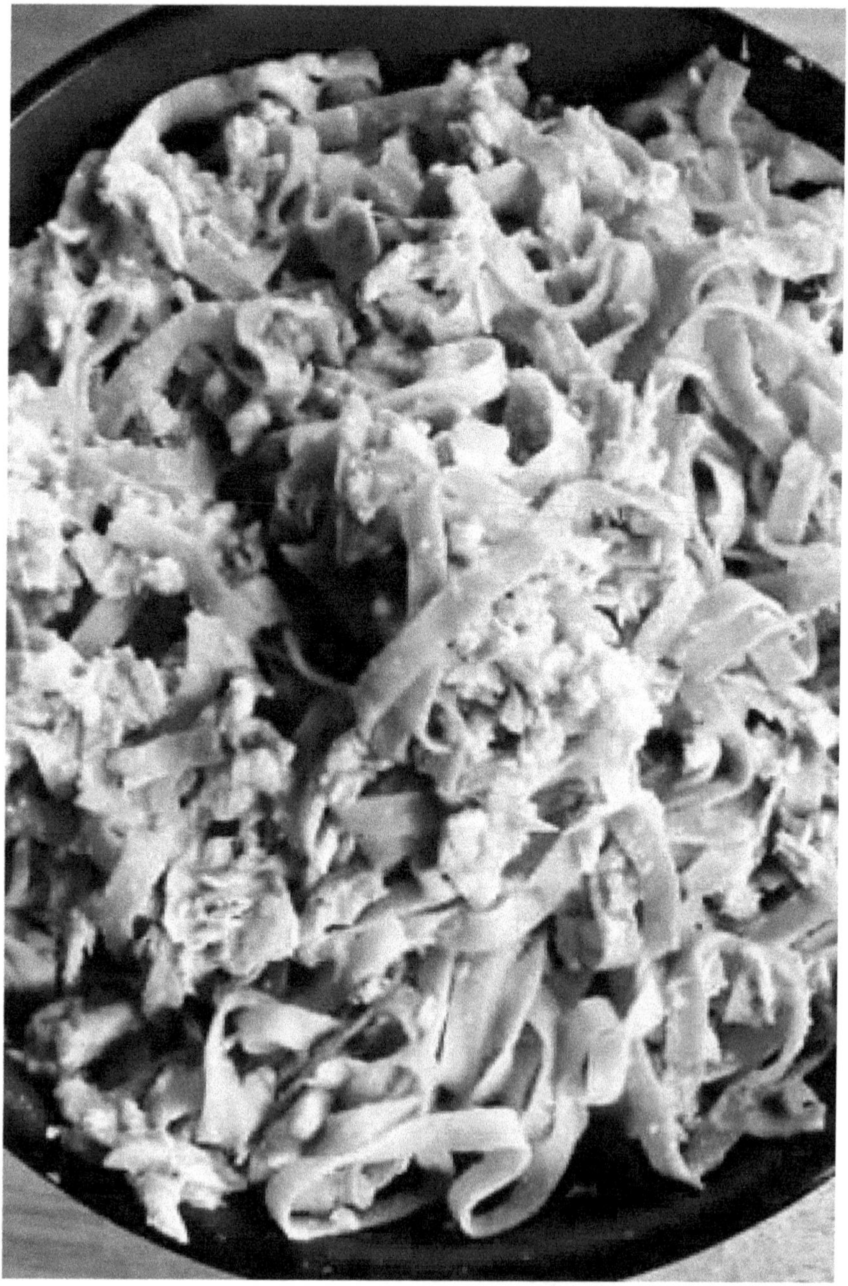

Tuna Salad Pickle Boats

Preparation Time : 10 minutes

Cooking Time : 0 minutes;

Servings : 2

Ingredients

- 4 dill pickles
- 4 oz of tuna, packed in water, drained
- ¼ of lime, juiced
- 4 tbsp. mayonnaise
- Seasoning:
- ¼ tsp salt
- 1/8 tsp ground black pepper
- ¼ tsp paprika
- 1 tbsp. mustard paste

Directions:

1. Prepare tuna salad and for this, take a medium bowl, place tuna in it, add lime juice, mayonnaise, salt, black pepper, paprika, and mustard and stir until mixed.
2. Cut each pickle into half lengthwise, scoop out seeds, and then fill with tuna salad.
3. Serve.

Nutrition :

308.5 Calories; 23.7 g Fats; 17 g Protein; 3.8 g Net Carb; 3.1 g Fiber;

Shrimp Deviled Eggs

Preparation Time : 5 minutes
Cooking Time : 0 minutes;

Servings : 2

Ingredients

- 2 eggs, boiled
- 2 oz shrimps, cooked, chopped
- ½ tsp tabasco sauce
- ½ tsp mustard paste
- 2 tbsp. mayonnaise
- Seasoning:
- 1/8 tsp salt
- 1/8 tsp ground black pepper

Directions:

1. Peel the boiled eggs, then slice in half lengthwise and transfer egg yolks to a medium bowl by using a spoon.
2. Mash the egg yolk, add remaining ingredients and stir until well combined.
3. Spoon the egg yolk mixture into egg whites, and then serve.

Nutrition:

210 Calories; 16.4 g Fats; 14 g Protein; 1 g Net Carb; 0.1 g Fiber;

Herb Crusted Tilapia

Preparation Time : 5 minutes

Cooking Time : 10 minutes;

Servings : 2

Ingredients

- 2 fillets of tilapia
- ½ tsp garlic powder
- ½ tsp Italian seasoning
- ½ tsp dried parsley
- 1/3 tsp salt
- Seasoning:
- 2 tbsp. melted butter, unsalted
- 1 tbsp. avocado oil

Directions:

1. Turn on the broiler and then let it preheat.
2. Meanwhile, take a small bowl, place melted butter in it, stir in oil and garlic powder until mixed, and then brush this mixture over tilapia fillets.
3. Stir together remaining spices and then sprinkle them generously on tilapia until well coated.
4. Place seasoned tilapia in a baking pan, place the pan under the broiler and then bake for 10 minutes until tender and golden, brushing with garlic-butter every 2 minutes.
5. Serve.

Nutrition:

520 Calories; 35 g Fats; 36.2 g Protein; 13.6 g Net Carb; 0.6 g Fiber;

Tuna Stuffed Avocado

Preparation Time : 5 minutes

Cooking Time : 0 minutes;

Servings : 2

Ingredients

- 1 medium avocado
- ¼ of a lemon, juiced
- 5-ounce tuna, packed in water
- 1 green onion, chopped
- 2 slices of turkey bacon, cooked, crumbled
- Seasoning:
- ¼ tsp salt
- ¼ tsp ground black pepper

Directions:

1. Drain tuna, place it in a bowl, and then broke it into pieces with a form.
2. Add remaining ingredients, except for avocado and bacon, and stir until well combined.
3. Cut avocado into half, remove its pit and then stuff its cavity evenly with the tuna mixture.
4. Top stuffed avocados with bacon and Serve.

Nutrition :

108.5 Calories; 8 g Fats; 6 g Protein; 0.8 g Net Carb; 2.3 g Fiber;

Garlic Butter Salmon

Preparation Time : 10 minutes

Cooking Time : 15 minutes

Servings : 2

Ingredients

- 2 salmon fillets, skinless
- 1 tsp minced garlic
- 1 tbsp. chopped cilantro
- 1 tbsp. unsalted butter
- 2 tbsp. grated cheddar cheese
- Seasoning:
- ½ tsp salt
- ¼ tsp ground black pepper

Directions:

1. Turn on the oven, then set it to 350 degrees F, and let it preheat.
2. Meanwhile, taking a rimmed baking sheet, grease it with oil, place salmon fillets on it, season with salt and black pepper on both sides.
3. Stir together butter, cilantro, and cheese until combined, then coat the mixture on both sides of salmon in an even layer and bake for 15 minutes until thoroughly cooked.
4. Then Turn on the broiler and continue baking the salmon for 2 minutes until the top is golden brown.
5. Serve.

Nutrition:

128 Calories; 4.5 g Fats; 41 g Protein; 1 g Net Carb; 0 g Fiber;

Salmon with Green Beans

Preparation Time : 10 minutes

Cooking Time : 20 minutes

Servings : 2

Ingredients

- 6 oz green beans
- 3 oz unsalted butter
- 2 salmon fillets
- Seasoning:
- ½ tsp garlic powder
- ½ tsp salt
- ½ tsp cracked black pepper

Directions:

1. Take a frying pan, place butter in it and when it starts to melts, add beans and salmon in fillets in it, season with garlic powder, salt, and black pepper, and cook for 8 minutes until salmon is cooked, turning halfway through and stirring the beans frequently.
2. When done, evenly divide salmon and green beans between two plates and serve.

Nutrition:

352 Calories; 29 g Fats; 19 g Protein; 3.5 g Net Carb; 1.5 g Fiber;

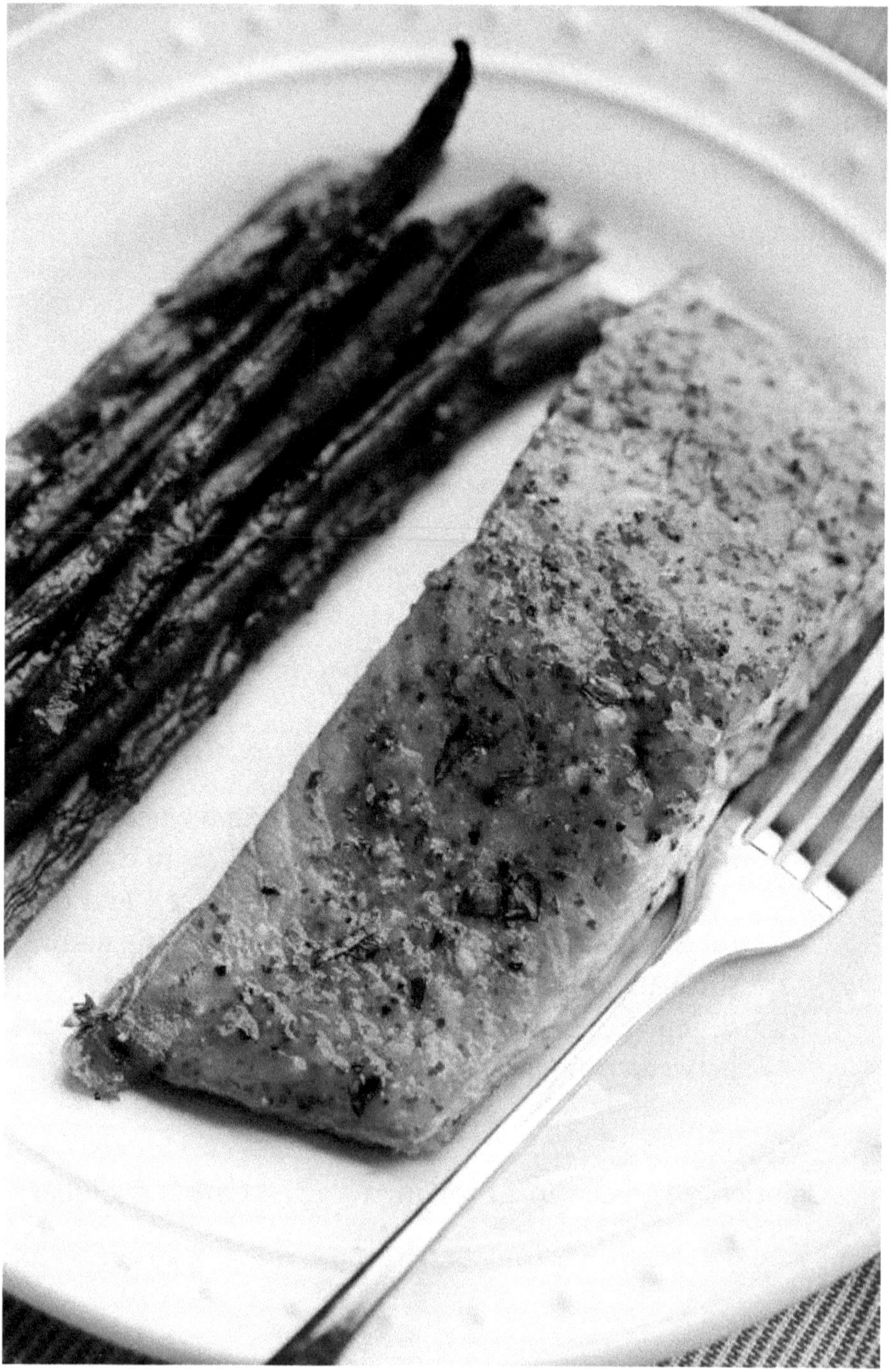

Salmon Sheet pan

Preparation Time : 10 minutes

Cooking Time : 20 minutes

Servings : 2

Ingredients

- 2 salmon fillets
- 2 oz cauliflower florets
- 2 oz broccoli florets
- 1 tsp minced garlic
- 1 tbsp. chopped cilantro
- Seasoning:
- 2 tbsp. coconut oil
- 2/3 tsp salt
- ¼ tsp ground black pepper

Directions:

1. Turn on the oven, then set it to 400 degrees F, and let it preheat.
2. Place oil in a small bowl, add garlic and cilantro, stir well, and microwave for 1 minute or until the oil has melted.
3. Take a rimmed baking sheet, place cauliflower and broccoli florets in it, drizzle with 1 tbsp. of coconut oil mixture, season with 1/3 tsp salt, 1/8 tsp black pepper and bake for 10 minutes.
4. Then push the vegetables to a side, place salmon fillets in the pan, drizzle with remaining coconut oil mixture, season with remaining salt and black pepper

on both sides and bake for 10 minutes until salmon is fork-tender.

5. Serve.

Nutrition :

450 Calories; 23.8 g Fats; 36.9 g Protein; 5.9 g Net Carb; 2.4 g Fiber;

Bacon wrapped Salmon

Preparation Time : 5 minutes
Cooking Time : 10 minutes

Servings : 2

Ingredients

- 2 salmon fillets, cut into four pieces
- 4 slices of bacon
- 2 tsp avocado oil
- 2 tbsp. mayonnaise
- Seasoning:
- ½ tsp salt
- ½ tsp ground black pepper

Directions:

1. Turn on the oven, then set it to 375 degrees F and let it preheat.
2. Meanwhile, place a skillet pan, place it over medium-high heat, add oil and let it heat.
3. Season salmon fillets with salt and black pepper, wrap each salmon fillet with a bacon slice, then add to the pan and cook for 4 minutes, turning halfway through.
4. Then transfer skillet pan containing salmon into the oven and cook salmon for 5 minutes until thoroughly cooked.
5. Serve salmon with mayonnaise

Nutrition:
190.7 Calories; 16.5 g Fats; 10.5 g Protein; 0 g Net Carb; 0 g Fiber;

Stir-fry Tuna with Vegetables

Preparation Time : 5 minutes;
Cooking Time : 15 minutes

Servings : 2

Ingredients

- 4 oz tuna, packed in water
- 2 oz broccoli florets
- ½ of red bell pepper, cored, sliced
- ½ tsp minced garlic
- ½ tsp sesame seeds
- Seasoning:
- 1 tbsp. avocado oil
- 2/3 tsp soy sauce
- 2/3 tsp apple cider vinegar
- 3 tbsp. water

Directions:

1. Take a skillet pan, add ½ tbsp. oil and when hot, add bell pepper and cook for 3 minutes until tender-crisp.
2. Then add broccoli floret, drizzle with water and continue cooking for 3 minutes until steamed, covering the pan.
3. Uncover the pan, cook for 2 minutes until all the liquid has evaporated, and then push bell pepper to one side of the pan.
4. Add remaining oil to the other side of the pan, add tuna and cook for 3 minutes until seared on all sides.

5. Then drizzle with soy sauce and vinegar, toss all the ingredients in the pan until mixed and sprinkle with sesame seeds.
6. Serve.

Nutrition:

99.7 Calories; 5.1 g Fats; 11 g Protein; 1.6 g Net Carb; 1 g Fiber;

Chili-glazed Salmon

Preparation Time : 5 minutes

Cooking Time : 10 minutes

Servings : 2

Ingredients

- 2 salmon fillets
- 2 tbsp. sweet chili sauce
- 2 tsp chopped chives
- ½ tsp sesame seeds

Directions:

1. Turn on the oven, then set it to 400 degrees F and let it preheat.
2. Meanwhile, place salmon in a shallow dish, add chili sauce and chives and toss until mixed.
3. Transfer prepared salmon onto a baking sheet lined with parchment sheet, drizzle with remaining sauce and bake for 10 minutes until thoroughly cooked.
4. Garnish with sesame seeds and Serve.

Nutrition:

112.5 Calories; 5.6 g Fats; 12 g Protein; 3.4 g Net Carb; 0 g Fiber;

Cardamom Salmon

Preparation Time : 5 minutes

Cooking Time : 20 minutes

Servings : 2

Ingredients

- 2 salmon fillets
- ¾ tsp salt
- 2/3 tbsp. ground cardamom
- 1 tbsp. liquid stevia
- 1 ½ tbsp. avocado oil

Directions:

1. Turn on the oven, then set it to 275 degrees F and let it preheat.
2. Meanwhile, prepare the sauce and for this, place oil in a small bowl, and whisk in cardamom and stevia until combined.
3. Take a baking dish, place salmon in it, brush with prepared sauce on all sides, and let it marinate for 20 minutes at room temperature.
4. Then season salmon with salt and bake for 15 to 20 minutes until thoroughly cooked.
5. When done, flake salmon with two forks and then serve.

Nutrition:

143.3 Calories; 10.7 g Fats; 11.8 g Protein; 0 g Net Carb; 0 g Fiber;

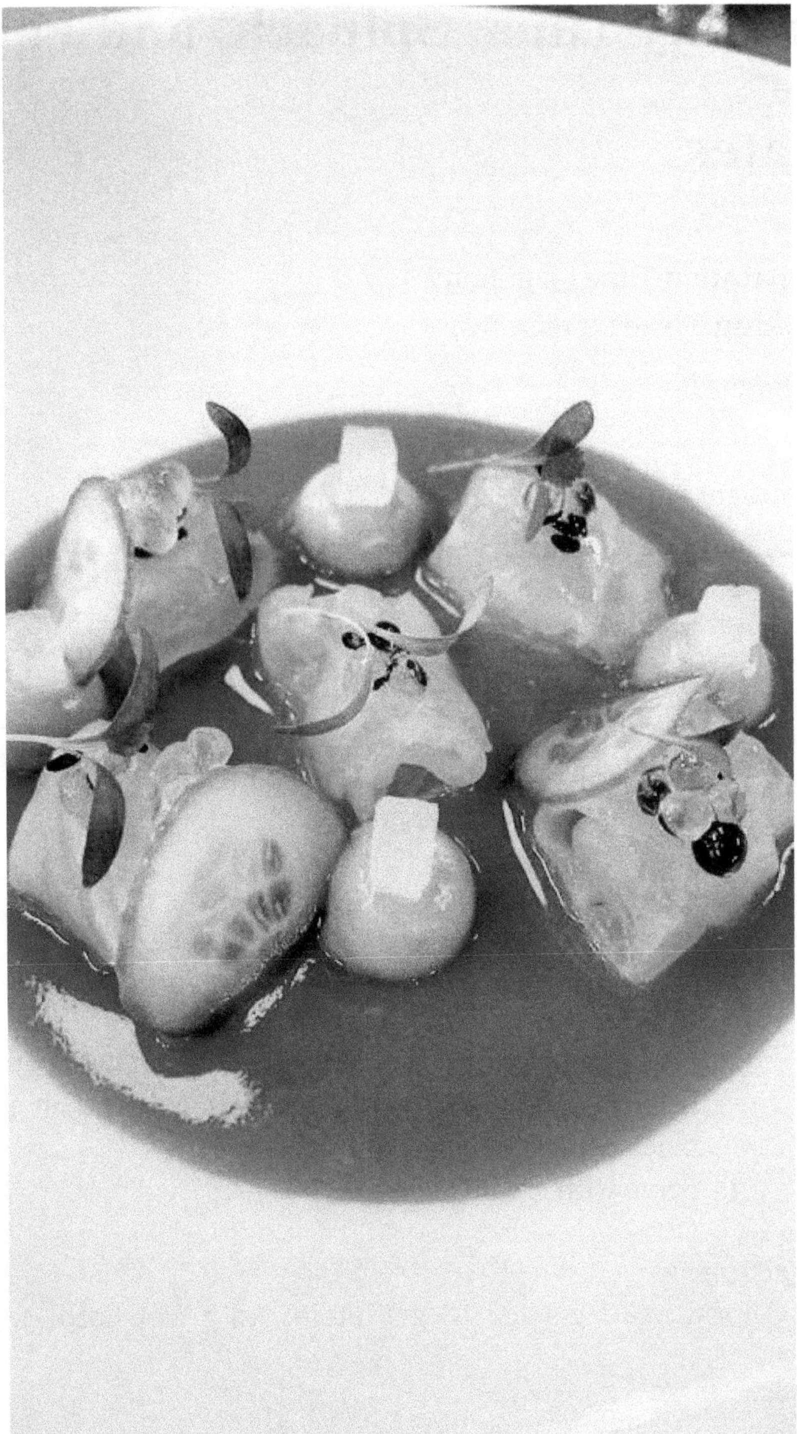

Creamy Tuna, Spinach, and Eggs Plates

Preparation Time : 5 minutes

Cooking Time : 0 minutes;

Servings : 2

Ingredients

- 2 oz of spinach leaves
- 2 oz tuna, packed in water
- 2 eggs, boiled
- 4 tbsp. cream cheese, full-fat
- Seasoning:
- ¼ tsp salt
- 1/8 tsp ground black pepper

Directions:

1. Take two plates and evenly distribute spinach and tuna between them.
2. Peel the eggs, cut them into half, and divide them between the plates and then season with salt and black pepper.
3. Serve with cream cheese.

Nutrition:

212 Calories; 14.1 g Fats; 18 g Protein; 1.9 g Net Carb; 1.3 g Fiber;

Tuna and Avocado

Preparation Time : 5 minutes;

Cooking Time : 0 minutes;

Servings : 2

Ingredients

- 2 oz tuna, packed in water
- 1 avocado, pitted
- 8 green olives
- ½ cup mayonnaise, full-fat
- Seasoning:
- 1/3 tsp salt
- 1/4 tsp ground black pepper

Directions:

1. Cut avocado into half, then remove the pit, scoop out the flesh and distribute between two plates.
2. Add tuna and green olives and then season with salt and black pepper.
3. Serve with mayonnaise.

Nutrition :
680 Calories; 65.6 g Fats; 10.2 g Protein; 2.2 g Net Carb; 9.7 g Fiber;

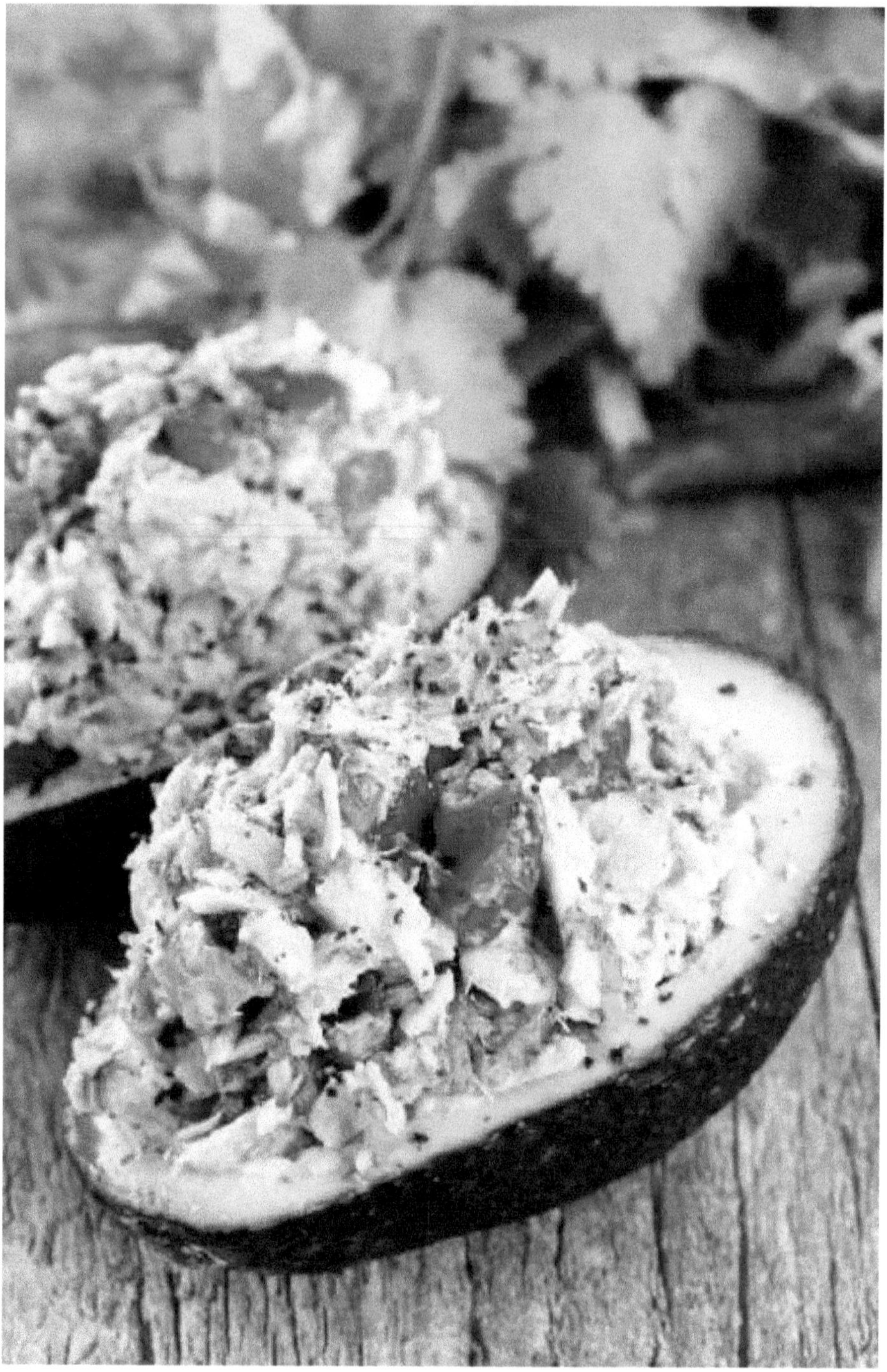

Baked Fish with Feta and Tomato

Preparation Time : 5 minutes
Cooking Time : 15 minutes;

Servings : 2

Ingredients

- 2 pacific whitening fillets
- 1 scallion, chopped
- 1 Roma tomato, chopped
- 1 tsp fresh oregano
- 1-ounce feta cheese, crumbled
- Seasoning:
- 2 tbsp. avocado oil
- 1/3 tsp salt
- 1/4 tsp ground black pepper
- ¼ crushed red pepper

Directions:

1. Turn on the oven, then set it to 400 degrees F and let it preheat.
2. Take a medium skillet pan, place it over medium heat, add oil and when hot, add scallion and cook for 3 minutes.
3. Add tomatoes, stir in ½ tsp oregano, 1/8 tsp salt, black pepper, red pepper, pour in ¼ cup water and bring it to simmer.

4. Sprinkle remaining salt over fillets, add to the pan, drizzle with remaining oil, and then bake for 10 to 12 minutes until fillets are fork-tender.
5. When done, top fish with remaining oregano and cheese and then serve.

Nutrition :

427.5 Calories; 29.5 g Fats; 26.7 g Protein; 8 g Net Carb; 4 g Fiber;

Garlic Oregano Fish

Preparation Time : 5 minutes
Cooking Time : 12 minutes;

Servings : 2

Ingredients

- 2 pacific whitening fillets
- 1 tsp minced garlic
- 1 tbsp. butter, unsalted
- 2 tsp dried oregano
- Seasoning:
- 1/3 tsp salt
- 1/4 tsp ground black pepper

Directions:

1. Turn on the oven, then set it to 400 degrees F and let it preheat.
2. Meanwhile, take a small saucepan, place it over low heat, add butter and when it melts, stir in garlic and cook for 1 minute, remove the pan from heat.
3. Season fillets with salt and black pepper, and place them on a baking dish greased with oil.
4. Pour butter mixture over fillets, then sprinkle with oregano and bake for 10 to 12 minutes until thoroughly cooked.
5. Serve.

Nutrition :

199.5 Calories; 7 g Fats; 33.5 g Protein; 0.9 g Net Carb; 0.1 g Fiber;

Fish and Spinach Plate

Preparation Time : 10 minutes
Cooking Time : 10 minutes;

Servings : 2

Ingredients

- 2 pacific whitening fillets
- 2 oz spinach
- ½ cup mayonnaise
- 1 tbsp. avocado oil
- 1 tbsp. unsalted butter
- Seasoning:
- 1/2 tsp salt
- 1/3 tsp ground black pepper

Directions:

1. Take a frying pan, place it over medium heat, add butter and wait until it melts.
2. Season fillets with 1/3 tsp salt and ¼ tsp black pepper, add to the pan, and cook for 5 minutes per side until golden brown and thoroughly cooked.
3. Transfer fillets to two plates, then distribute spinach among them, drizzle with oil and season with remaining salt and black pepper.
4. Serve with mayonnaise.

Nutrition :

389 Calories; 34 g Fats; 7.7 g Protein; 10.6 g Net Carb; 2 g Fiber

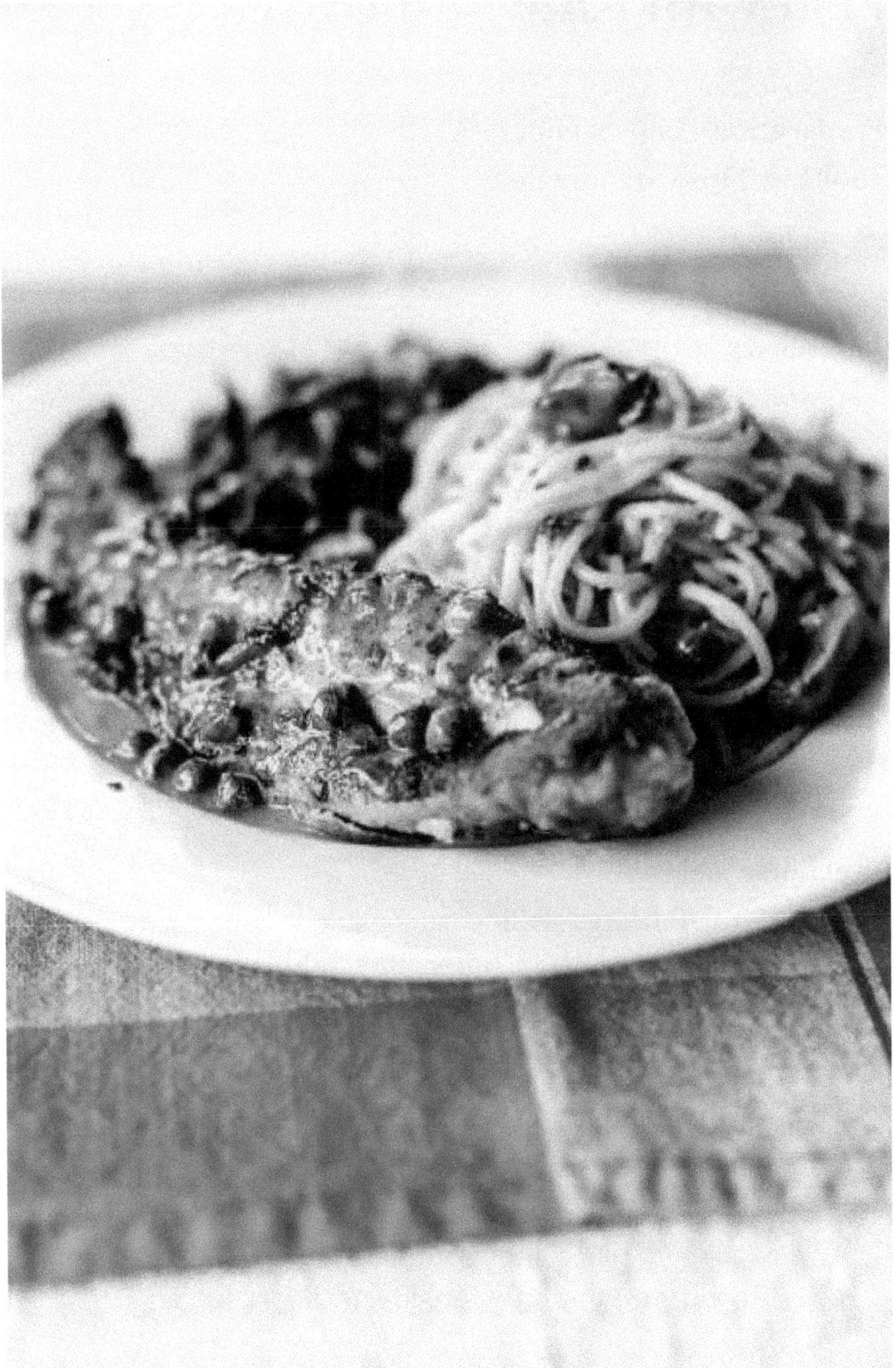

Fish with Kale and Olives

Preparation Time : 5 minutes

Cooking Time : 12 minutes;

Servings : 2

Ingredients

- 2 pacific whitening fillets
- 2 oz chopped kale
- 3 tbsp. coconut oil
- 2 scallion, chopped
- 6 green olives
- Seasoning:
- 1/2 tsp salt
- 1/3 tsp ground black pepper
- 3 drops of liquid stevia

Directions:

1. Take a large skillet pan, place it over medium-high heat, add 4 tbsp. water, then add kale, toss and cook for 2 minutes until leaves are wilted but green.
2. When done, transfer kale to a strainer placed on a bowl and set aside until required.
3. Wipe clean the pan, add 2 tbsp. oil, and wait until it melts.
4. Season fillets with 1/3 tsp salt and ¼ tsp black pepper, place them into the pan skin-side up and cook for 4 minutes per side until fork tender.

5. Transfer fillets to a plate, add remaining oil to the pan, then add scallion and olives and cook for 1 minute.
6. Return kale into the pan, stir until mixed, cook for 1 minute until hot and then season with remaining salt and black pepper.
7. Divide kale mixture between two plates, top with cooked fillets, and then serve.

Nutrition:
454 Calories; 35.8 g Fats; 16 g Protein; 13.5 g Net Carb; 3.5 g Fiber;

Mahi-Mahi with Chili Lime Butter

Preparation Time : 5 minutes
Cooking Time : 10 minutes;

Servings : 2

Ingredients

- 3 tbsp. coconut oil, divided
- ½ tsp red chili powder
- 2 mahi-mahi fillets
- 1 lime, zested
- Seasoning:
- 1/3 tsp salt
- ¼ tsp ground black pepper

Directions:

1. Prepare the chili-lime butter and for this, take a small bowl, add 2 tbsp. coconut oil in it and then stir in red chili powder and lime zest until combined, set aside until required.
2. Take a medium skillet pan, place it over medium-high heat, add remaining oil and wait until it melts.
3. Season fillets with salt and black pepper, add to the pan and cook for 5 minutes per side until thoroughly cooked and golden brown.

4. When done, transfer fillets to the plates, top generously with prepared chili-lime butter, and then serve.

Nutrition:
298 Calories; 18.2 g Fats; 31.5 g Protein; 0.1 g Net Carb; 0.2 g Fiber;

Ginger Sesame Glazed Salmon

Preparation Time : 10 minutes;

Cooking Time : 15 minutes;

Servings : 2

Ingredients

- 2 salmon fillets
- 1 tbsp. soy sauce
- 1 tsp sesame oil
- 2 tsp fish sauce
- 1 tbsp. avocado oil
- Seasoning:
- 1 tsp garlic powder
- 1 tsp ginger powder
- ½ tbsp. apple cider vinegar

Directions:

1. Prepare the marinade and for this, take a small bowl, place soy sauce in it and stir in sesame oil, fish sauce, sesame oil, avocado oil, vinegar, ginger powder and garlic powder and stir until mixed.
2. Place salmon fillets in a shallow dish, pour prepared marinate on it, toss until coated, and let it marinate for 10 minutes.
3. When ready to cook, take a griddle pan, place it over medium heat, grease it with oil, and when hot, place marinated salmon fillets on it and then grill for 5 to 7 minutes per side until done.

4. Serve.

Nutrition:

370 Calories; 23.5 g Fats; 33 g Protein; 2.5 g Net Carb; 0 g Fiber

Tuna, Dill and Spinach Curry Bowl

Preparation Time : 5 minutes
Cooking Time : 0 minutes;

 Servings : 2

Ingredients

- 3 oz tuna, packed in water
- 1 green onion, sliced
- 1 tbsp. diced dill pickle
- 1/3 of avocado, sliced
- 1 ounce chopped spinach
- Seasoning:
- 1 ½ tsp curry powder
- ¼ tsp of sea salt
- 5 tbsp. mayonnaise

Directions:

1. Take a medium bowl, place mayonnaise in it, and then stir in curry powder and salt.
2. Add tuna, onion, dill pickle and spinach, toss until well coated, and then top with avocado.
3. Serve.

Nutrition :

310 Calories; 28 g Fats; 12.2 g Protein; 1 g Net Carb; 0.5 g Fiber;

Mushroom with Salmon

Preparation Time : 5 minutes
Cooking Time : 15 minutes;

Servings : 2

Ingredients

- 2 salmon fillets
- 2 oz sliced mushrooms
- 1 tbsp. avocado oil
- 3 tbsp. butter, unsalted
- ¼ cup of water
- Seasoning:
- 3/4 tsp salt
- 1/2 tsp ground black pepper
- ¼ tsp paprika

Directions:

1. Take a medium skillet pan, place it over medium heat, add oil and wait until it gets hot.
2. Season salmon with ½ tsp salt and ¼ tsp black pepper, add them to the pan and cook for 3 minutes per side until brown, set aside until done.
3. Add 2 tbsp. butter into the pan and when it melts, add mushrooms, season with paprika and remaining salt and black pepper, and cook for 3 minutes until sauté.
4. Pour in water, stir well, then add remaining butter and when it melts, return pork chops into the pan and simmer for 3 minutes until cooked.

5. Serve.

Nutrition :

420 Calories; 34.2 g Fats; 25 g Protein; 1.8 g Net Carb; 0.3 g Fiber;

Tuna Salad Cucumber Boats

Preparation Time : 10 minutes
Cooking Time : 0 minutes;

Servings : 2

Ingredients

- 1 cucumber
- 2 oz tuna, packed in water
- 1 green onion, sliced
- 2 1/2 tbsp. mayonnaise
- 1 tsp mustard paste
- Seasoning:
- ¼ tsp salt
- 1/8 tsp ground black pepper

Directions:

1. Prepare salad and for this, place tuna in a bowl, add onion, mayonnaise and mustard, then add salt and black pepper and stir until combined.
2. Cut cucumber from the middle lengthwise, then scrape out the inside by using a spoon and fill the space with tuna salad.
3. Serve.

Nutrition:

190 Calories; 14.2 g Fats; 8.8 g Protein; 3.6 g Net Carb; 2 g Fiber;

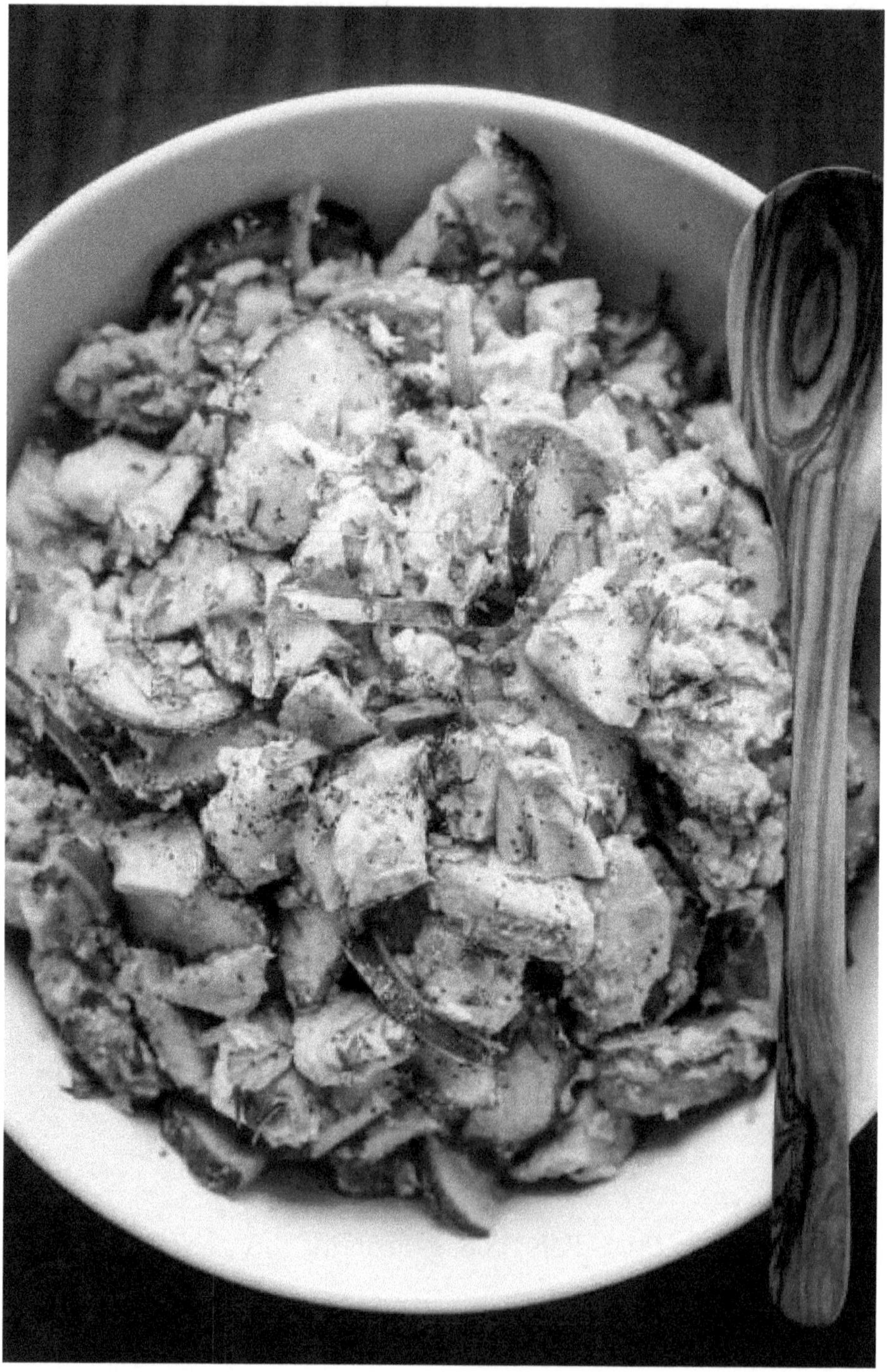

Salmon with Lime Butter Sauce

Preparation Time : 20 minutes

Cooking Time : 10 minutes;

Servings : 2

Ingredients

- 2 salmon fillets
- 1 lime, juiced, divided
- ½ tbsp. minced garlic
- 3 tbsp. butter, unsalted
- 1 tbsp. avocado oil
- Seasoning:
- 1/4 tsp salt
- 1/4 tsp ground black pepper

Directions:

1. Prepare the fillets and for this, season fillets with salt and black pepper, place them on a shallow dish, drizzle with half of the lime juice and then it marinate for 15 minutes.
2. Meanwhile, prepare the lime butter sauce and for this, take a small saucepan, place it over medium-low heat, add butter, garlic, and half of the lime juice, stir until mixed, and then bring it to a low boil, set aside until required.
3. Then take a medium skillet pan, place it over medium-high heat, add oil and when hot, place marinated salmon in it, cook for 3 minutes per side and then transfer to a plate.

4. Top each salmon with prepared lime butter sauce and then serve.

Nutrition:
192 Calories; 18 g Fats; 6 g Protein; 4 g Net Carb; 0 g Fiber;

Blackened Fish with Zucchini Noodles

Preparation Time : 10 minutes;
Cooking Time : 12 minutes;

Servings : 2

Ingredients

- 1 large zucchini
- 2 fillets of mahi-mahi
- 1 tsp Cajun seasoning
- 2 tbsp. butter, unsalted
- 1 tbsp. avocado oil
- Seasoning:
- ½ tsp garlic powder
- 2/3 tsp salt
- ½ tsp ground black pepper

Directions:

1. Spiralized zucchini into noodles, place them into a colander, sprinkle with 1/3 tsp salt, toss until mixed and set aside until required.
2. Meanwhile, prepare fish and for this, season fillets with remaining salt and ¾ tsp Cajun seasoning.
3. Take a medium skillet pan, place it over medium heat, add butter and when it melts, add prepared fillets, switch heat to medium-high level and cook for

3 to 4 minutes per side until cooked and nicely browned.

4. Transfer fillets to a plate and then reserve the pan for zucchini noodles.
5. Squeeze moisture from the noodles, add them to the skillet pan, add oil, toss until mixed, season with remaining Cajun seasoning and cook for 2 to 3 minutes until noodles have turned soft.
6. Sprinkle with garlic powder, remove the pan from heat and distribute noodles between two plates.
7. Top noodles with a fillet and then serve.

Nutrition :

350 Calories; 25 g Fats; 27.1 g Protein; 2.8 g Net Carb; 1.6 g Fiber;

Garlic Parmesan Mahi-Mahi

Preparation Time : 10 minutes
Cooking Time : 10 minutes;

Servings : 2

Ingredients

- 2 fillets of mahi-mahi
- 1 tsp minced garlic
- 1/3 tsp dried thyme
- 1 tbsp. avocado oil
- 1 tbsp. grated parmesan cheese
- Seasoning:
- 1/3 tsp salt
- 1/4 tsp ground black pepper

Directions:

1. Turn on the oven, set it to 425 degrees F and let it preheat.
2. Meanwhile, take a small bowl, place oil in it, add garlic, thyme, cheese and oil and stir until mixed.
3. Season fillets with salt and black pepper, then coat with prepared cheese mixture, place fillets in a baking sheet and then cook for 7 to 10 minutes until thoroughly cooked.
4. Serve.

Nutrition:

170 Calories; 7.8 g Fats; 22.3 g Protein; 0.8 g Net Carb; 0 g Fiber;

Salmon with Roasted Veggies

Preparation Time : 10 minutes

Cooking Time : 15 minutes;

Servings : 2

Ingredients

- 2 fillets of salmon
- 4 oz asparagus spears cut
- 2 oz sliced mushrooms
- 2 oz grape tomatoes
- 2 oz basil pesto
- Seasoning:
- 2/3 tsp salt
- ½ tsp ground black pepper
- 1 tbsp. mayonnaise
  - oz grated mozzarella cheese
- 2 tbsp. avocado oil

Directions:

2. Turn on the oven, then set it to 425 degrees F and let it preheat.
3. Take a medium baking sheet lined with parchment paper, place salmon fillets on it and then season with 1/3 tsp salt and ¼ tsp ground black pepper.
4. Take a small bowl, mix together mayonnaise and pesto in it until combined, spread this mixture over seasoned salmon and then top evenly with cheese.

5. Take a medium bowl, place all the vegetables in it, season with remaining salt and black pepper, drizzle with oil and toss until coated.
6. Spread vegetables around prepared fillets and then bake for 12 to 15 minutes until fillets have thoroughly cooked.
7. Serve.

Nutrition:
571 Calories; 45.4 g Fats; 34.1 g Protein; 3.5 g Net Carb; 2.2 g Fiber;

Cheesy Baked Mahi-Mahi

Preparation Time : 10 minutes

Cooking Time : 25 minutes;

Servings : 2

Ingredients

- 2 fillets of mahi-mahi
- ½ tsp minced garlic
- 2 tbsp. mayonnaise
- 1 tbsp. grated parmesan cheese
- 1 tbsp. grated mozzarella cheese
- Seasoning:
- ½ tsp salt
- ¼ tsp ground black pepper
- 1 tbsp. mustard paste
- ¼ of lime, juiced

Directions:

1. Turn on the oven, then set it to 400 degrees F and let it preheat.
2. Meanwhile, take a baking sheet, line it with foil, place fillets on it and then season with salt and black pepper.
3. Take a small bowl, add mayonnaise, stir in garlic, lime juice and mustard until well mixed and then spread this mixture evenly on fillets.
4. Stir together parmesan cheese and mozzarella cheese, sprinkle it over fillets and then bake for 15 to 20 minutes until thoroughly cooked.

5. Then Turn on the broiler and continue cooking the fillets for 2 to 3 minutes until the top is nicely golden brown.
6. Serve.

Nutrition :
241 Calories; 13.6 g Fats; 25 g Protein; 1.1 g Net Carb; 0 g Fiber;

Zucchini Noodles in Creamy Salmon Sauce

Preparation Time : 5 minutes;
Cooking Time : 7 minutes;

Servings : 2

Ingredients

- 3 oz smoked salmon
- 1 zucchini, spiralized into noodles
- 1 tbsp. chopped basil
- 2 oz whipping cream
- 2 oz cream cheese, softened
- Seasoning:
- 1/3 tsp salt
- 1/3 tsp ground black pepper
- 1 tbsp. avocado oil

Directions:

1. Cut zucchini into noodles, place them into a colander, sprinkle with some salt, toss until well coated and set aside for 10 minutes.
2. Meanwhile, take a small saucepan, place it over medium-low heat, add whipped cream in it, add cream cheese, stir until mixed, bring it to a simmer, and cook for 2 minutes or more until smooth.
3. Then switch heat to low heat, add basil into the pan, cut salmon into thin slices, add to the pan, season

with ¼ tsp of each salt and black pepper and cook for 1 minute until hot, set aside until required.

4. Take a medium skillet pan, place it over medium-high heat, add oil and when hot, add zucchini noodles and cook for 1 to 2 minutes until fried.
5. Season zucchini with remaining salt and black pepper and then distribute zucchini between two plates.
6. Top zucchini noodles with salmon sauce and then serve.

Nutrition :

271 Calories; 22 g Fats; 13.5 g Protein; 4.5 g Net Carb; 1.5 g Fiber;

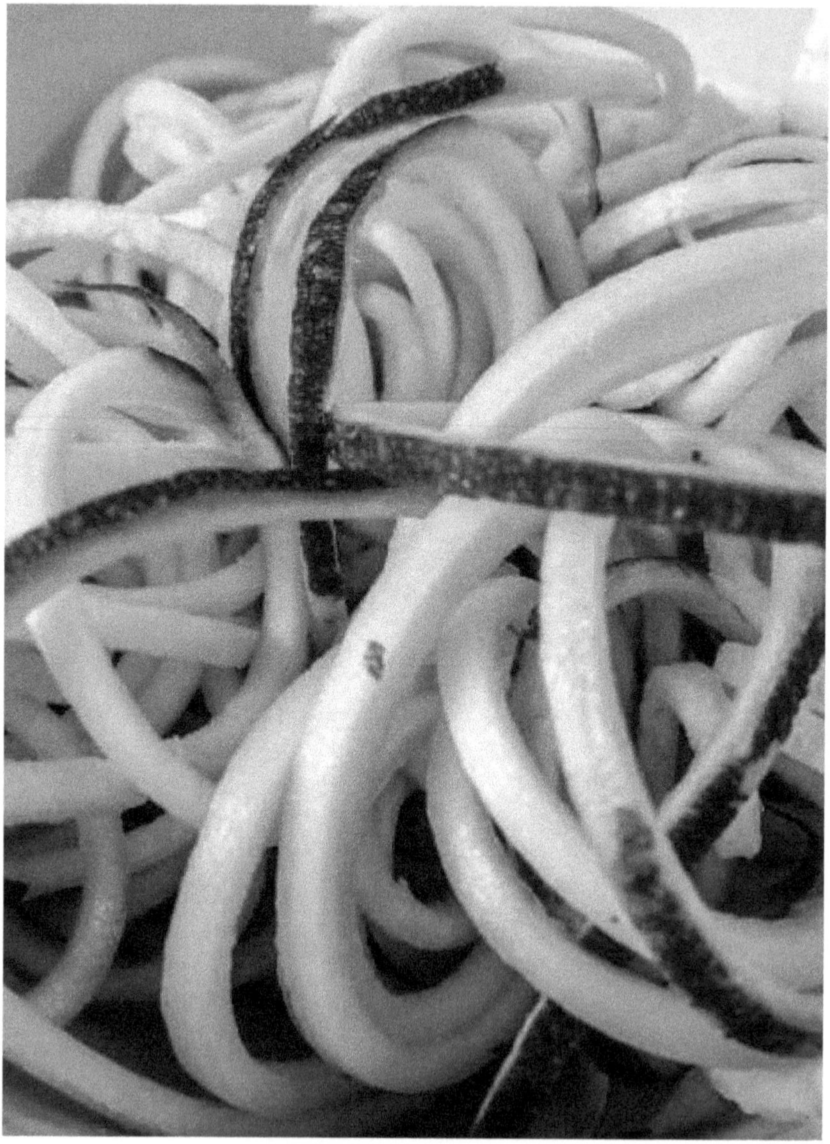

Winter Comfort stew

Preparation Time: 15 minutes

Cooking Time: 50 minutes

Servings: 6

Ingredients:

- 2 tbsp. olive oil
- 1 small yellow onion, chopped
- 2 garlic cloves, chopped
- 2 lb. grass-fed beef chuck, cut into 1-inch cubes
- 1 (14-oz.) can sugar-free crushed tomatoes
- 2 tsp. ground allspice
- 1½ tsp. red pepper flakes
- ½ C. homemade beef broth
- 6 oz. green olives, pitted
- 8 oz. fresh baby spinach
- 2 tbsp. fresh lemon juice
- Salt and freshly ground black pepper, to taste
- ¼ C. fresh cilantro, chopped

Direction:

1. In a pan, heat the oil in a pan over high heat and sauté the onion and garlic for about 2-3 minutes.
2. Add the beef and cook for about 3-4 minutes or until browned, stirring frequently.
3. Add the tomatoes, spices and broth and bring to a boil.

4. Reduce the heat to low and simmer, covered for about 30-40 minutes or until desired doneness of the beef.
5. Stir in the olives and spinach and simmer for about 2-3 minutes.
6. Stir in the lemon juice, salt and black pepper and remove from the heat.
7. Serve hot with the garnishing of cilantro.

Nutrition:

Calories: 388; Carbohydrates: 8g; Protein: 485g; Fat: 17.7g; Sugar: 2.6g; Sodium: 473mg; Fiber: 3.1g

Ideal Cold Weather Stew

Preparation Time: 20 minutes

Cooking Time: 2 hours 40 minutes

Servings: 6

Ingredients:

- 3 tbsp. olive oil, divided
- 8 oz. fresh mushrooms, quartered
- 1¼ lb. grass-fed beef chuck roast, trimmed and cubed into 1-inch size
- 2 tbsp. tomato paste
- ½ tsp. dried thyme
- 1 bay leaf
- 5 C. homemade beef broth
- 6 oz. celery root, peeled and cubed
- 4 oz. yellow onions, chopped roughly
- 3 oz. carrot, peeled and sliced
- 2 garlic cloves, sliced
- Salt and freshly ground black pepper, to taste

Direction:

1. In a Dutch oven, heat 1 tbsp. of the oil over medium heat and cook the mushrooms for about 2 minutes, without stirring.
2. Stir the mushroom and cook for about 2 minutes more.
3. With a slotted spoon, transfer the mushroom onto a plate.

4. In the same pan, heat the remaining oil over medium-high heat and sear the beef cubes for about 4-5 minutes.
5. Stir in the tomato paste, thyme and bay leaf and cook for about 1 minute.
6. Stir in the broth and bring to a boil.
7. Reduce the heat to low and simmer, covered for about 1½ hours.
8. Stir in the mushrooms, celery, onion, carrot and garlic and simmers for about 40-60 minutes.
9. Stir in the salt and black pepper and remove from the heat.
10. Serve hot.

Nutrition:

Calories: 447; Carbohydrates: 7.4g; Protein: 30.8g; Fat: 32.3g; Sugar: 8g; Sodium: 764mg; Fiber: 1.9g

Weekend Dinner Stew

Preparation Time: 15 minutes

Cooking Time: 55 minutes

Servings: 6

Ingredients:

- 1½ lb. grass-fed beef stew meat, trimmed and cubed into 1-inch size
- Salt and freshly ground black pepper, to taste
- 1 tbsp. olive oil
- 1 C. homemade tomato puree
- 4 C. homemade beef broth
- 2 C. zucchini, chopped
- 2 celery ribs, sliced
- ½ C. carrots, peeled and sliced
- 2 garlic cloves, minced
- ½ tbsp. dried thyme
- 1 tsp. dried parsley
- 1 tsp. dried rosemary
- 1 tbsp. paprika
- 1 tsp. onion powder
- 1 tsp. garlic powder

Direction:

1. In a large bowl, add the beef cubes, salt and black pepper and toss to coat well.

2. In a large pan, heat the oil over medium-high heat and cook the beef cubes for about 4-5 minutes or until browned.
3. Add the remaining ingredients and stir to combine.
4. Increase the heat to high and bring to a boil.
5. Reduce the heat to low and simmer, covered for about 40-50 minutes.
6. Stir in the salt and black pepper and remove from the heat.
7. Serve hot.

Nutrition:

Calories: 293; Carbohydrates: 8g; Protein: 9.3g; Fat: 10.7g; Sugar: 4g; Sodium: 223mg; Fiber: 2.3g

Mexican Pork Stew

Preparation Time: 15 minutes

Cooking Time: 2 hours 10 minutes

Servings: 1

Ingredients:

- 3 tbsp. unsalted butter
- 2½ lb. boneless pork ribs, cut into ¾-inch cubes
- 1 large yellow onion, chopped
- 4 garlic cloves, crushed
- 1½ C. homemade chicken broth
- 2 (10-oz.) cans sugar-free diced tomatoes
- 1 C. canned roasted poblano chiles
- 2 tsp. dried oregano
- 1 tsp. ground cumin
- Salt, to taste
- ¼ C. fresh cilantro, chopped
- 2 tbsp. fresh lime juice

Direction:

1. In a large pan, melt the butter over medium-high heat and cook the pork, onions and garlic for about 5 minutes or until browned.
2. Add the broth and scrape up the browned bits.
3. Add the tomatoes, poblano chiles, oregano, cumin, and salt and bring to a boil.
4. Reduce the heat to medium-low and simmer, covered for about 2 hours.

5. Stir in the fresh cilantro and lime juice and remove from heat.
6. Serve hot.

Nutrition:

Calories: 288; Carbohydrates: 8.8g; Protein: 39.6g; Fat: 10.1g; Sugar: 4g; Sodium: 283mg; Fiber: 2.8g

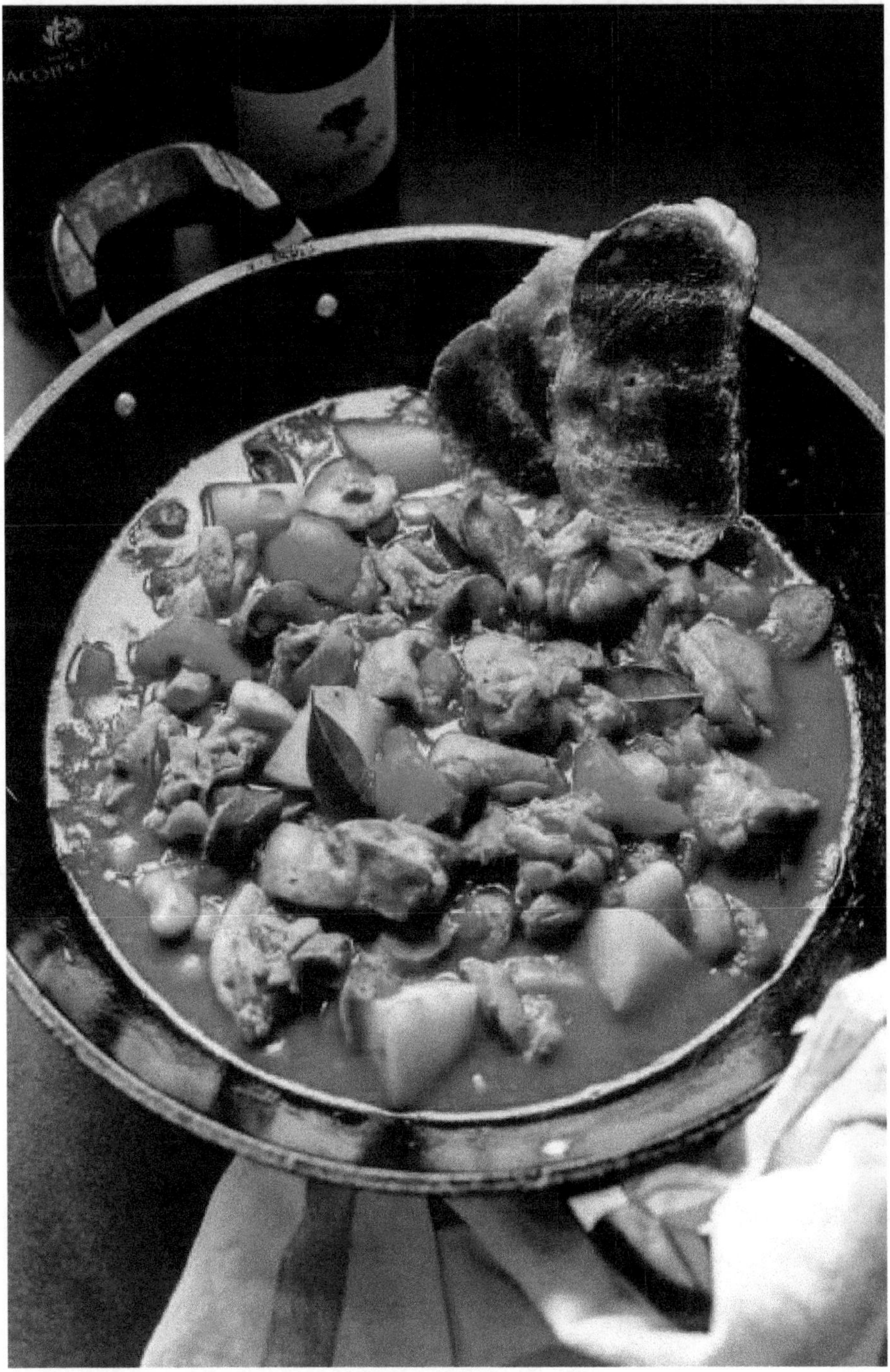

Hungarian Pork Stew

Preparation Time: 15 minutes

Cooking Time: 2 hours 20 minutes

Servings: 10

Ingredients:

- 3 tbsp. olive oil
- 3½ lb. pork shoulder, cut into 4 portions
- 1 tbsp. butter
- 2 medium onions, chopped
- 16 oz. tomatoes, crushed
- 5 garlic cloves, crushed
- 2 Hungarian wax peppers, chopped
- 3 tbsp. Hungarian Sweet paprika
- 1 tbsp. smoked paprika
- 1 tsp. hot paprika
- ½ tsp. caraway seeds
- 1 bay leaf
- 1 C. homemade chicken broth
- 1 packet unflavored gelatin
- 2 tbsp. fresh lemon juice
- Pinch of xanthan gum
- Salt and freshly ground black pepper, to taste

Directions:

1. In a heavy-bottomed pan, heat 1 tbsp. of oil over high heat and sear the pork for about 2-3 minutes or until browned.

2. Transfer the pork onto a plate and cut into bite-sized pieces.
3. In the same pan, heat 1 tbsp. of oil and butter over medium-low heat and sauté the onions for about 5-6 minutes.
4. With a slotted spoon transfer the onion into a bowl.
5. In the same pan, add the tomatoes and cook for about 3-4 minutes, without stirring.
6. Meanwhile, in a small frying pan, heat the remaining oil over-low heat and sauté the garlic, wax peppers, all kinds of paprika and caraway seeds for about 20-30 seconds.
7. Remove from the heat and set aside.
8. In a small bowl, mix together the gelatin and broth.
9. In the large pan, add the cooked pork, garlic mixture, gelatin mixture and bay leaf and bring to a gentle boil.
10. Reduce the heat to low and simmer, covered for about 2 hours.
11. Stir in the xanthan gum and simmer for about 3-5 minutes.
12. Stir in the lemon juice, salt and black pepper and remove from the heat.
13. Serve hot.

Nutrition:

Calories: 529; Carbohydrates: 5.8g; Protein: 38.9g; Fat: 38.5g; Sugar: 2.6g; Sodium: 216mg; Fiber: 2.1g

Yellow Chicken Soup

Preparation Time: 15 minutes

Cooking Time: 25 minutes

Servings: 5

Ingredients:

- 2½ tsp. ground turmeric
- 1½ tsp. ground cumin
- 1/8 tsp cayenne pepper
- 2 tbsp. butter, divided
- 1 small yellow onion, chopped
- 2 C. cauliflower, chopped
- 2 C. broccoli, chopped
- 4 C. homemade chicken broth
- 1½ C. water
- 1 tsp. fresh ginger root, grated
- 1 bay leaf
- 2 C. Swiss chard, stemmed and chopped finely
- ½ C. unsweetened coconut milk
- 3 (4-oz.) grass-fed boneless, skinless chicken thighs, cut into bite-size pieces
- 2 tbsp. fresh lime juice

Direction:

1. In a small bowl, mix together the turmeric, cumin and cayenne pepper and set aside.
2. Ina large pan, melt 1 tbsp. of the butter over medium heat and sauté the onion for about 3-4 minutes.

3. Add the cauliflower, broccoli and half of the spice mixture and cook for another 3-4 minutes.
4. Add the broth, water, ginger and bay leaf and bring to a boil.
5. Reduce the heat to low and simmer for about 8-10 minutes.
6. Stir in the Swiss chard and coconut milk and cook for about 1-2 minutes.
7. Meanwhile, in a large skillet, melt the remaining butter over medium heat and sear the chicken pieces for about 5 minutes.
8. Stir in the remaining spice mix and cook for about 5 minutes, stirring frequently.
9. Transfer the soup into serving bowls and top with the chicken pieces.
10. Drizzle with lime juice and serve.

Nutrition:

Calories: 258; Carbohydrates: 8.4g; Protein: 18.4g; Fat: 16.8g; Sugar: 3g; Sodium: 753mg; Fiber: 2.9g

Curry Soup

Preparation Time: 25 minutes

Cooking Time: 20 minutes

Servings: 4

Ingredients:

- ¾ tsp. cumin
- ¼ c. pumpkin seeds, raw
- ½ tsp. garlic powder
- ½ tsp. paprika ½ tsp. sea salt
- 1 c. coconut milk, unsweetened
- 1 clove garlic, minced
- 1 med. onion, diced
- 2 c. carrots, chopped
- 2 tbsp. curry powder
- 3 c. cauliflower, riced
- 3 tbsp. extra virgin olive oil, divided
- 4 c. kale, chopped
- 4 c. vegetable broth
- Sea salt & pepper to taste

Direction:

1. Hear a large saute pan over medium heat with 2 tablespoons of olive oil. Once the oil is hot, add the rice cauliflower to the pan along with the curry powder, cumin, salt, paprika, and garlic powder. Stir thoroughly to combine.
2. While cooking, stir occasionally. Once the cauliflower is warmed through, remove it from the heat.

3. In a large pot over medium heat, add the remainder of your olive oil. Once it's hot, add the onion and allow it to cook for about four minutes. Add the garlic, then cook for about another two minutes.
4. To the large pot, add the broth, kale, carrots, and cauliflower. Stir to incorporate thoroughly.
5. Allow the mixture to come to a boil, drop the heat to low, and allow the soup to simmer for about 15 minutes.
6. Stir the coconut milk into the mixture along with salt and pepper to taste.
7. Garnish with pumpkin seeds and serve hot!

Nutrition:

Calories: 274; Carbs: 11 grams; Fat: 19 grams; Protein: 15 grams

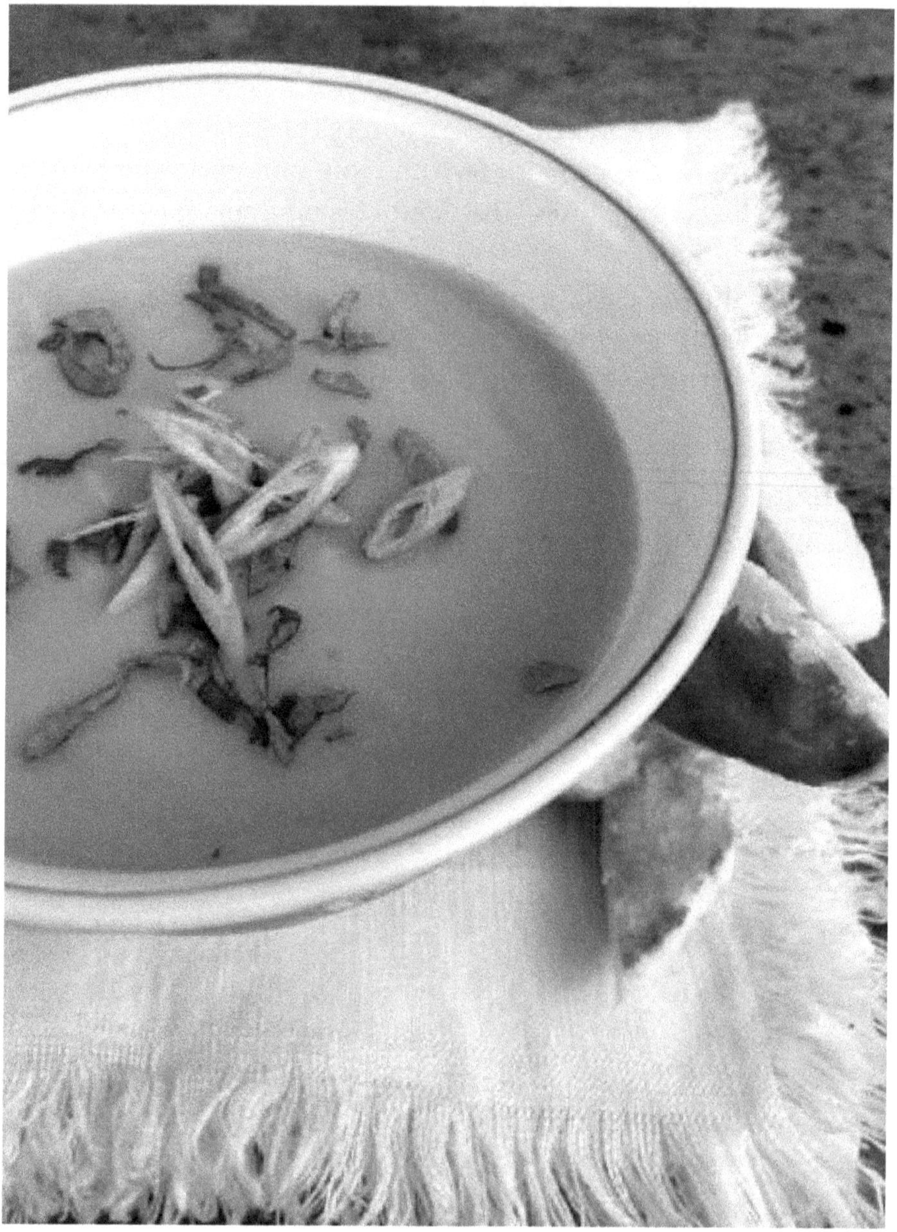

Delicious Tomato Basil Soup

Preparation Time: 10 minutes

Cooking Time: 40 minutes

Servings: 4

Ingredients:
- ¼ c. olive oil
- ½ c. heavy cream
- 1 lb. tomatoes, fresh
- 4 c. chicken broth, divided
- 4 cloves garlic, fresh
- Sea salt & pepper to taste

Direction:
1. Preheat oven to 400° Fahrenheit and line a baking sheet with foil.
2. Remove the cores from your tomatoes and place them on the baking sheet along with the cloves of garlic.
3. Drizzle tomatoes and garlic with olive oil, salt, and pepper.
4. Roast at 400° Fahrenheit for 30 minutes.
5. Pull the tomatoes out of the oven and place into a blender, along with the juices that have dripped onto the pan during roasting.
6. Add two cups of the chicken broth to the blender.
7. Blend until smooth, then strain the mixture into a large saucepan or a pot.

8. While the pan is on the stove, whisk the remaining two cups of broth and the cream into the soup.
9. Simmer for about ten minutes.
10. Season to taste, then serve hot!

Nutrition:

Calories: 225; Carbohydrates: 5.5 grams; Fat: 20 grams; Protein: 6.5 grams

30-Day Meal Plan

Days	Breakfast	Lunch	Dinner	Snacks
1	Bacon Cheeseburger Waffles	Buttered Cod	Baked Crispy Chicken	Fluffy Bites
2	Keto Breakfast Cheesecake	Salmon with Red Curry Sauce	Italian Chicken	Coconut Fudge
3	Egg-Crust Pizza	Salmon Teriyaki	Chicken & Carrots	Nutmeg Nougat
4	Breakfast Roll Ups	Pesto Shrimp with Zucchini Noodles	Lemon & Herb Chicken	Sweet Almond Bites
5	Basic Opie Rolls	Crab Cakes	Chicken & Avocado Salad	Strawberry Cheesecake Minis
6	Cream Cheese Pancake	Tuna Salad	Chicken Bowl	Cocoa Brownies
7	Blueberry Coconut Porridge	Keto Frosty	Chicken with Bacon & Ranch Sauce	Chocolate Orange Bites
8	Cauliflower Hash Browns	Keto Shake	Creamy Chicken & Mushroo	Caramel Cones

			m	
9	**Keto Rolls**	Keto Fat Bombs	Mozzarella Chicken	Cinnamon Bites
10	**Breakfast Roll Ups**	Avocado Ice Pops	Chicken Parmesan	Sweet Chai Bites
11	**Almond Flour Pancakes**	Carrot Balls	Pasta	Easy Vanilla Bombs
12	**Avocado Toast**	Coconut Crack Bars	Crab Melt	Marinated Eggs.
13	**Chicken Avocado Egg Bacon Salad**	Strawberry Ice Cream	Spinach Frittata	Sausage and Cheese Dip.
14	**Bacon Wrapped Chicken Breast**	Key Lime Pudding	Halloumi Time	Tasty Onion and Cauliflower Dip.
15	**Egg Salad**	Easy Meatballs	Hash Browns	Pesto Crackers.
16	**Blueberry Muffins**	Chicken in Sweet and Sour Sauce with Corn Salad	Poblano Peppers	Pumpkin Muffins.
17	**Bacon Hash**	Chinese Chicken Salad	Mushroom Omelet	Cheesy Salami Snack
18	**Bagels With Cheese**	Chicken Salad	Tuna Casserole	Creamy Mango and Mint Dip
19	**Cauli Flitters**	Tofu Meat and Salad	Goat Cheese	Hot Red Chili and

			Frittata	Garlic Chutney
20	**Scrambled Eggs**	Asparagus and Pistachios Vinaigrette	Pasta	Red Chilies and Onion Chutney
21	**Frittata with Spinach**	Turkey Meatballs	Muffins	Fast Guacamole
22	**Cheese Omelet**	Easy Meatballs	Meaty Salad	Coconut Dill Dip
23	**Capicola Egg Cups**	Chicken, Bacon and Avocado Cloud Sandwiches	Pasta	Creamy Crab Dip
24	**Breakfast Roll Ups**	Roasted Lemon Chicken Sandwich	Crab Soup	Creamy Cheddar and Bacon Spread with Almonds
25	**Overnight "noats"**	Keto-Friendly Skillet Pepperoni Pizza	Southern Bean Casserole	Green Tabasco Devilled Eggs
26	**Frozen keto coffee**	Cheesy Chicken Cauliflower	Low-Carb Okra	Herbed Cheese Balls
27	**Easy Skillet Pancakes**	Chicken Soup	Cauli Rice	Cheesy Salami Snack
28	**Quick Keto**	Chicken	Southern	Pesto &

	Blender Muffins	Avocado Salad	Fried Chicken	Olive Fat Bombs
29	**Keto Everything Bagels**	Chicken Broccoli Dinner	Low-Carb Lasagna	Cheesy Broccoli Nuggets
30	**Turmeric Chicken and Kale Salad with Food, Lemon and Honey**	Easy Meatballs	Low-Carb Spaghetti Bolognese	Salmon Fat Bombs

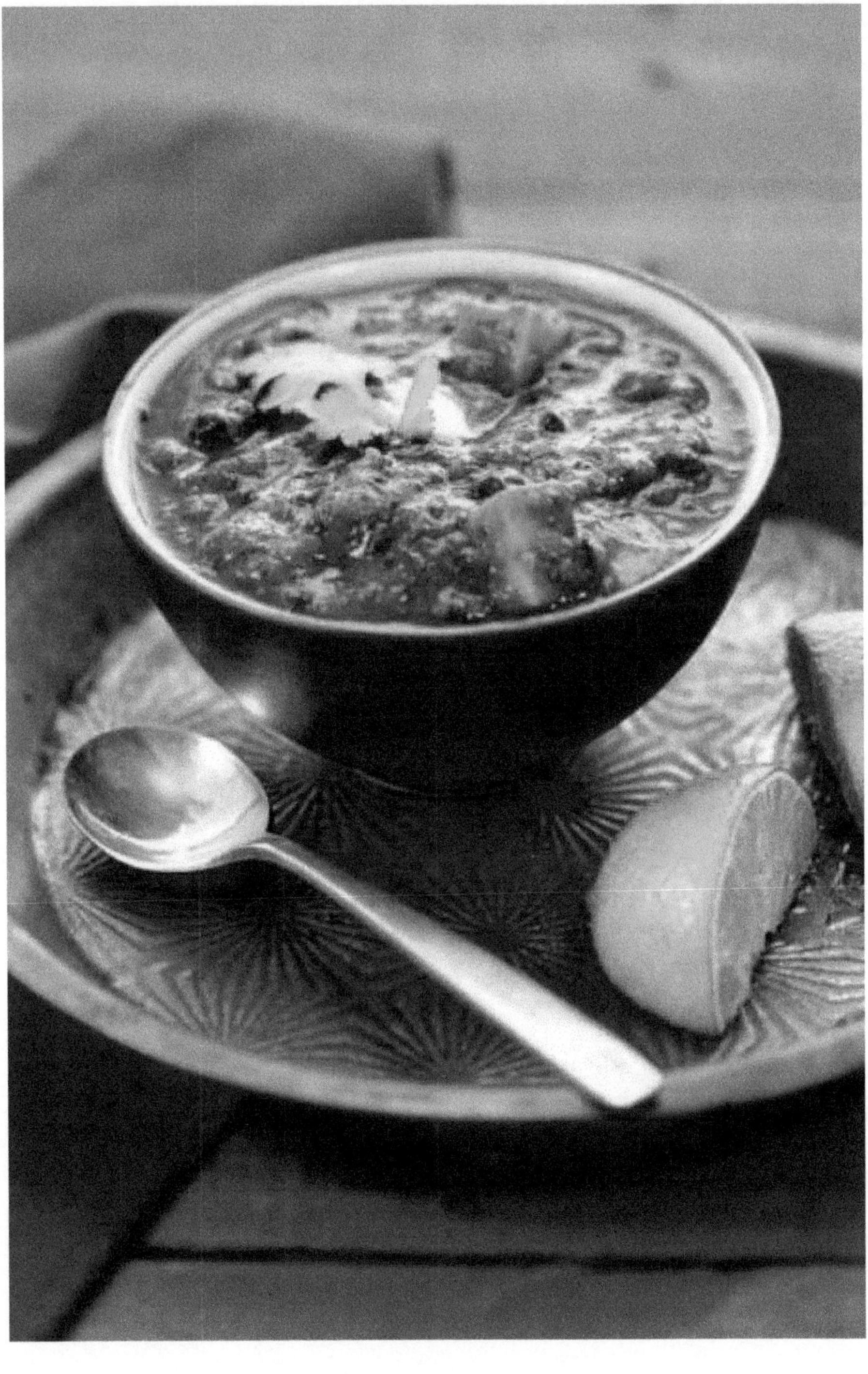

Lightning Source UK Ltd.
Milton Keynes UK
UKHW020801230621
386011UK00006B/36

9 781802 779073